"This book could be a godsend for anyone suffering from lifelong issues around eating, weight, and appearance. It presents a sane and novel approach to finding a balanced relationship to food, eating, and your body through mindfulness. The book is written by someone with obvious depth of experience and savvy who is definitely on your side, whatever your difficulties or challenges. *Eat, Drink, and Be Mindful* may be just what the doctor ordered, or would have but couldn't—until now."

—Jon Kabat-Zinn, Ph.D., author of *Full Catastrophe Living, Arriving at Your Own Door,* and *Coming to Our Senses*

"*Eat, Drink, and Be Mindful* will jumpstart your new journey to a healthier life. We each make over 200 mindless eating decisions each day. By using the tips, exercises, and checklists in this book, you can make many of these 200 decisions work for you rather than against you. Albers' insights and personalized approach will inspire change and lead to more balance in your food life and your daily living."

—Brian Wansink, Ph.D., professor and director of Cornell University Food and Brand Lab and author of *Mindless Eating*

"*Eat, Drink, and be Mindful* is a compassionate, step-by-step workbook to help the diet-weary reader make peace with food, mind, and body. You'll discover your inner eating expert—you!—while putting an end to the inner food fight once and for all."

—Evelyn Tribole, MS, RD, nutrition therapist and coauthor of *Intuitive Eating*

"Whether or not you struggle with food or weight, this book is for you! *Eat, Drink, and Be Mindful* promises to make a real difference in people's lives. All will be nourished and touched by the wisdom it carries."

—Jenni Schaefer, author of *Life Without Ed*

"Albers' wonderful new book, *Eat, Drink, and Be Mindful,* is one of the best workbooks I have seen on the subject of mindful eating. It could prove to be a very worthwhile choice for all those struggling with mindless eating habits. Her book is extremely well organized and very easy to use. It is a very practical, nonjudgmental, and useful manual on how to eat and drink in awareness. A great follow-up workbook to use with her first book, *Eating Mindfully.*"

—Jeanie Seward-Magee, BSW, Mindful Way course presenter and author of *A Mindful Way*

"*Eat, Drink and Be Mindful* provides you with simple, realistic changes that you can make today to improve your health and well-being. With this book, America is one step closer to mindfully changing its eating habits!"

> —James O. Hill, Ph.D., professor of pediatrics at the University of Colorado, Denver, and author of T*he Step Diet Book*

"*Eat, Drink, and be Mindful* is a must-read for anyone who struggles with healthy eating in our fast-paced, weight-obsessed society. Albers's approach is kind, compassionate, and a breath of fresh air. I will recommend this book to all my clients, graduate students, colleagues, and friends."

> —Kathleen Burns Kingsbury, LMHC, CPCC, president of KBK Connections, Inc., and coauthor of *Weight Wisdom*

"*Eat, Drink, and Be Mindful* is an inviting, valuable, and user-friendly guide for using mindfulness in the vital, everyday activities of eating and nourishing your body. Susan Albers's easy-to-follow mindfulness practices and suggestions provide readers with a direct pathway to greater joy, greater wisdom, and better health. Moreover, practicing mindful eating can restore a sense of presence and richness to each moment that will permeate every aspect of your life."

> —Jeffrey Brantley, MD, founder and director of the mindfulness-based stress reduction program at Duke Integrative Medicine, Duke University, Durham, NC, and author of *Calming Your Anxious Mind*

eat, drink, and be mindful

how to end your struggle
with mindless eating and
start savoring food with
intention and joy

susan albers, psy.d.

New Harbinger Publications, Inc.

Distributed in Canada by Raincoast Books

New Harbinger Publications, Inc.
5674 Shattuck Avenue
Oakland, CA 94609
www.newharbinger.com

Cover design by Amy Shoup; Text design by Amy Shoup and Michele Waters-Kermes; Acquired by Catharine Sutker; Edited by Karen O'Donnell Stein

Library of Congress Cataloging-in-Publication Data

Albers, Susan, Psy.D.
    Eat, drink, and be mindful : how to end your struggle with mindless eating and start savoring food with intention and joy / Susan Albers.
        p. cm.
    Includes bibliographical references.
    ISBN-13: 978-1-57224-615-7 (pbk. : alk. paper)
    ISBN-10: 1-57224-615-4 (pbk. : alk. paper) 1. Food habits--Psychological aspects. 2. Nutrition--Psychological aspects. 3. Eating (Philosophy) 4. Awareness. I. Title.
    TX357.A393 2008
    613.2--dc22

                                          2008039797

12   11   10

10   9   8   7   6   5   4   3   2

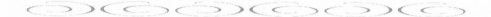

This workbook is dedicated to
my clients and readers
who requested a workbook,
and to
Brooklyn V. Bowling

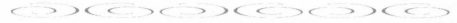

contents

online resources 189

references 191

acknowledgments

One cannot think well, love well,
sleep well, if one has not dined well.
—Virginia Woolf

Thank you for the professional input and influence of Susan Heady, Dr. Trey Hill, Dr. Jason Greif, Dr. Luis G. Manzo, Dr. Victoria Gould, and the staff and doctors at the Cleveland Clinic Women's Health Center.

Thanks to my good friends: Jane Lindquist Lesniewski, Betsy Beyer Swope, Eric Lingenfelter, Bronwyn Wilke Lingenfelter, and Victoria Gould.

My best to John R. Bowling; Carmela and Thomas Albers; Angie Albers; Linda, Judd, Paul, and Jenna Serotta; and John, Rhonda, and Jim Bowling.

I appreciate the support and assistance of the New Harbinger editors and staff, who made this project possible.

I would like to send a special thank-you to Natalie Murphy. Her contributions were an invaluable addition to this book. I appreciate her enthusiasm for mindful eating.

introduction

Let me begin by telling you a story. When my first book, *Eating Mindfully,* was first released to bookstores, I began receiving e-mails from people all over the world—from Montana to Chile to Japan. Hundreds of people wrote to me about their struggles with mindless eating. Some of the men and women had just recently developed eating issues, and others had been dealing with eating problems for more than forty years. I was touched by each story. Every letter made me more mindful of how painful and difficult mindless-eating issues can be.

As grateful as I was for these readers' willingness to share their stories, curiosity got the better of me. I wondered how readers had learned about *Eating Mindfully.* There are so many weight management resources available; how were readers led to this particular book? So I took an informal survey. Many people had gotten the book from a doctor or a friend. Or they had read an excerpt in a magazine or newspaper like *O, the Oprah Magazine; Natural Health; Self;* or the *Wall Street Journal.* However, the majority of people responded that they had discovered the book while they were on a quest for a quick fix. While looking for books on the Atkins diet, they happened upon my book (books by Atkins and Albers are often right next to each other on the shelf, because they both begin with *A*). Maybe they tried Dr. Atkins's diet, but when that didn't work, they turned to *Eating Mindfully.*

Dr. Atkins would probably have a thing or two to say about mindful eating if he were still alive. Mindful eating, in many ways, is very different from the Atkins diet. The Atkins diet generally involves cutting out certain types of foods. In contrast, rather than making certain foods strictly off-limits, mindful eating is about balancing your diet, gaining awareness of your mindless-eating habits, and tailoring your approach to your body's needs. Thankfully, the high-protein, low-carbohydrate diet craze is slowing down. But the newest, greatest diet is surely just around the corner. So, if dieting hasn't worked for you or if you have started a diet and ended it in the same day, that is okay. Mindful eating will stick around for good. Diets come and go like the latest fashions, but mindful eating is a lifelong approach to healthy eating that includes all foods.

Mindful eating is also helpful for people who have deeper struggles with food. People who undereat, overeat, binge, or have a chaotic relationship with food can use this approach as well. Unlike alcoholics, who work on cutting out alcohol from their lives, people who have a significant problem with food must still come in contact with the substance that is so troubling to them every single day, at least three times a day. This gives mindless eaters two very big tasks to master: First, they need to learn how to avoid using food to regulate their feelings. Second, they must get adequate food and nutrients without overdoing or underdoing it. This workbook is one resource that can help you develop the tools to do both of these tasks.

Perhaps you read *Eating Mindfully* and hoped for another practical tool that would assist you on your journey toward mindful eating. Numerous colleagues, clients, and readers requested just such a workbook. For this reason, I created this workbook, which is intended to be interactive: it's a journal to help raise your awareness, and it can also be used to document your progress. If you have no experience with this approach, that's okay; this book is for beginners as well as more-advanced mindful eaters.

As you work your way through the book, you'll find, as many of my colleagues and clients have, that mindful eating has many advantages over dieting. Below, you'll find a list of some of the rewards my clients have experienced from this approach.

ten benefits of mindful eating

Let's take a look at some of the many benefits of mindful eating.

1. **It's a non-diet approach.** Fad diets don't work. We like to think that they do, but they don't. Diets appear to be effective because people often lose weight at first. However, 95 percent of all dieters regain the lost weight and gain more within one to five years (Grodstein et al. 1996). Worst of all, diets warp your relationship with food. They are a significant trigger of disordered eating and eating disorders. Fad diets teach you not to trust your body. Lose-weight-quick schemes tell you to just ignore your hunger. Mindful eating is about creating balance and appropriately responding to your body's needs.

2. **It's not scary.** Let's face it, eating issues are hard! Many people aren't afraid of mindful eating because it is a nonjudgmental approach. There aren't strict rules that make you feel like a bad person if you don't (or can't) follow them. You can go at your own pace and tailor your eating to your needs.

3. **The exercises are realistic and doable.** A lot of programs are just too cumbersome and time consuming. Or, the plan orders you to eat foods that aren't really part of your regular diet, like cabbage, or only meats.

4. **It advocates self-acceptance and body acceptance.** Do you find yourself thinking, "I'd feel better about myself if I ate healthier or managed my weight, but I need to feel better about myself to get the motivation to eat better"? This is why accepting yourself as you are now is key.

5. **It lasts.** It provides tools that will stay with you your entire life.

6. **It's nonjudgmental and compassionate.** Self-criticism has never helped anyone adapt his or her behavior. Understanding and encouragement create the right environment for change.

7. **It works!** Research shows that mindfulness helps you gain more control of your eating habits (Proulx 2008; Smith et al. 2006). For this reason, it is a great long-term approach for managing your weight.

8. **It's holistic.** Mindful eating examines all dimensions of eating (mind, body, thoughts, and feelings).

9. **It's for everybody.** It is great for men and women, and for overeaters, undereaters, chaotic eaters, and dieters.

10. **It provides clarity.** Eating-disorder treatment professionals and nutritionists often instruct people not to diet. But in the same breath they advise, "However, don't just eat whatever you want." This is a conflicting message. These professionals clearly define what not to do, but they are less clear on what you should do. Eating mindfully brings clarity to this conflict. It tells you what *to do* rather than what *not to do*.

who is this workbook for?

Have you tried every diet imaginable?

Do you struggle with your weight?

Do you eat when you aren't even hungry?

Do you feel uncomfortable in your body or clothes?

Does your weight affect your health or well-being?

Does your weight ever stop you from doing fun things you want to do?

If you answered yes to any of these questions, this book is for you! But, really, this book is intended to be for everyone. Let me rephrase that: this book is for anyone who is seriously committed to being in charge of his or her eating habits and relationship with food, whether he or she is just starting out or has practiced for a long time. Even the most mindful eater can use a tune-up every now and then. Dealing with stress or being served special dishes during the holidays, such as pecan pie and sugar cookies, can make the most mindful eater slip.

If the mindless-eating symptoms listed in this book sound familiar to you, it's no cause for surprise. Mindless eating is a common problem. In fact, over 60 percent of Americans are classified as overweight or obese (DiBonaventura and Chapman 2008). For some people, the way they eat is a chronic problem; it causes problems in their day-to-day lives and is potentially dangerous. These people say that they can hardly remember what it was like to have a healthy relationship with food. Others may have fairly healthy eating habits but just need a guide to help them get back on track when they fall into mindless eating.

Like many people, you may have found yourself coming back to the problem of mindless eating again and again. It's hard to get off of the "why" merry-go-round.

getting off the "why" merry-go-round

You're on the "why" merry-go-round if you find yourself asking the following questions: "*Why* do I have these eating problems?" "*Why* has this been a struggle for me and not for other people?" "What *caused* the mindless eating issues?"

Yes, it is definitely important to know the factors that started the eating issues in the first place. However, many people find that they get stuck on the "why" merry-go-round. They go around and around asking the same question: "What caused this problem in the first place?" There might be some plausible answers. Perhaps you are genetically predisposed to have weight problems. Maybe your entire family has wrestled with obesity and body image. Maybe you got teased about your weight as a child. Perhaps you grew up in a controlling family and food was the only thing your parents couldn't take over in your life. There are so many possibilities!

Because there is no clear-cut answer, pursuing the "why" question can become a daunting and frustrating task. At some point, you will have to accept that you may never know for sure why your eating issues developed. You may have an idea of the root causes. However, continuing to get to the bottom of it may not be the answer. If you are stuck asking why, it doesn't help you to move on. Eventually, you will need some tools to fix the problem.

So, this brings you to your first lesson in acceptance, one of the seven skills of mindful eating: to accept that eating is a struggle for you, no matter how this struggle started. You have picked up this book, so it's likely that you've already accepted it on some level. That's a great start. Accepting that mindless eating is an issue even though you don't want it to be a problem—this is a big step that will help you get past the dead-end questions. This is the goal of the workbook: to help you get off the "why" merry-go-round and get you on the "how to" path.

how to use this workbook

Let's get started. You may wish to begin by carefully reading the rest of the introduction, particularly if you are new to the concept of mindful eating. It will give you the basic overview. Once you have done that, the only things you need are a pen and some time set aside to work through this book. That can be a challenge, but it's well worth the time and effort. Complete the self-assessments sprinkled throughout the book. They will ask you a lot of questions about your current and past habits, and they will help you get a sense of which chapters in the book to focus on, specifically the information that will be most helpful to you.

In chapter 2 you will read about the seven skills of becoming a mindful eater. Each of these skills will be discussed in the opening of a subsequent chapter. Each chapter will explain why that skill is an essential part of mindful eating and will expand on the skill in more detail. You'll find a variety of practical mindful eating exercises along the way. The exercises will help you incorporate mindful eating into your everyday life.

There are two types of exercises offered in this book. The first type features reflective questions, which help stimulate you to think deeply about your habits. It's important to write down the answers to these questions. Like keeping a diary or journal, writing helps you organize your thoughts, and reading your entries later gives you new insights. The second type of exercise is experiential. In these exercises, you will be putting mindful eating into practice with real-world challenges. For this reason, you may want to practice the skills in a variety of different contexts. Try the exercise once at breakfast and then again at dinner. Do the exercise at home and also at a restaurant. Eating is such a big part of our everyday lives that there are so many different opportunities to use this method.

Like learning any new skill, it takes time. Be patient. The more you practice, the better at it you will become. Of course, if you have been eating the same way for ten years, you aren't going to undo that habit overnight. But hang in there. It is possible! You may wish to take this workbook with you wherever you go so that you remember to use it. It's particularly helpful to open it up before and after mealtimes and anytime you notice yourself snacking mindlessly.

Another strategy is to read through the entire book and then go back and do the exercises. This may help you get the big picture before diving into the specifics. The format of the workbook is intended for you to write directly in it. Don't hesitate to mark up this book! To supplement your progress, you may wish to read *Eating Mindfully,* of which this workbook is an extension. *Eating Mindfully* discusses the concepts and skills in more detail. If you are a college student, you may wish to pick up *Mindful Eating 101: A Guide to Healthy Eating in College and Beyond,* which offers mindful eating tips for students who eat in cafeterias, battle exam stress, and cope with a variety of academic pressures.

The book was written with the intent of helping everyone learn the joys of mindful eating, no matter who you are or where you live. For this reason, you can use the workbook on your own, in therapy, or in a support group. If the workbook is recommended by a therapist, you'll find it helpful to buy your own copy so that you can write in it directly.

Once you've mastered the art of mindful eating, you may find yourself pulling this workbook out again in the future. Depending on the circumstances in your life or the time of year—such as during holidays or times when your weight has fluctuated—you may need a mini refresher. That's okay. This workbook is meant to help you at every step along the way.

where to find treatment and support

Many of my clients mention how helpful it is to have support and guidance from a professional. Keep in mind that this workbook is not intended as a substitute for therapy or advice from a medical professional. I would strongly recommend that you work closely with a group of treatment providers such as a therapist, psychologist, registered dietitian, nutritionist, and physician. If you have very problematic eating, start by bringing this workbook to a well-respected professional. It can be used as an adjunct to whatever kind of treatment you seek. Your therapist or doctor may help you to identify the parts of the workbook that will be most helpful to you.

My clients tell me that a few things held them back from taking the step to call a professional. Sometimes they were stuck on the fear that there might be a stigma associated with having mental health and eating issues. Thankfully, this is an outdated notion. Many people today are very aware of the mind-body connection. Those who still worry about this issue are concerned that people will think they are crazy or weak. I want to reassure you that this is quite the contrary! It is a healthy move to gather the best resources possible. If you were diabetic, would you decide to try to cure it on your own? No. You'd gather the right professionals to help you recover. The same goes for eating problems.

Another hurdle is the challenge of finding the right professional. Finding a specialist is a key issue, because each person's eating issues are unique and must be treated on a case-by-case basis. However, there are many ways to find great treatment. Here are a few places to start:

1. Check out www.edreferral.com. On this excellent site, you can click on your state and find treatment providers in your area. Professionals listed on this site have indicated that they have additional training or expertise with eating issues.

2. If you are looking for a nutrition professional, you can look on www.eatright.org, which offers information on how to find a professional near your hometown.

3. Contact the National Eating Disorders Association at 1-800-931-2237 or www.nationaleating disorders.org for information on how to find a nutritionist, support group, or mental health professional, such as a psychologist or doctor.

4. Ask a professional you trust, such as your doctor or a respected mental health organization. It's important to get a good recommendation. Feel free to call and interview the professional to see if he or she is a good match for your issues, and to make sure you feel comfortable with the person you will be working with. Once you've met with the professional, he or she can help you develop a plan that includes mindful eating. Bring along the workbook and work through it together.

how professionals can use this book

If you are like most mental health professionals and physicians, one of your greatest challenges is to find a book that you can confidently recommend to your patients and clients. You are looking for something that clients will actually read from start to finish. So many books are too long or too complicated; if they look too daunting, clients are too intimidated to even pick them up. You are seeking a book that provides much more detail than you are able to give clients during their limited session time with you. Most important, you are looking for a book that is positive, wellness focused, and sensitive. If you work with patients with eating issues, you are well aware of the shame and embarrassment patients carry inside them. You want to show your patients the best care and support you possibly can, which will be reflected in the literature you give to them to read.

This book is all of these things. For this reason, it is a great tool to use with clients. The workbook format allows clients to record their eating habits; you can ask them to keep a detailed record in the space provided and then review it with them in the office. In addition, the text clearly explains new skills for coping with problematic eating and offers exercises that are concise and easy for clients to use.

You'll notice that the workbook can be useful for the full range of eating problems, from everyday mindless eating to chronic mindless overeating and undereating problems. It covers the mind, body, and emotional issues that may be interfering with healthy eating habits. In this way, it helps you address eating issues from many different angles.

Mindful Eating Support Groups

A support group can easily use this text. The one-topic-per-chapter format lends itself well to covering a particular issue each week. Group members can be given weekly assignments, and they can then use the mindful eating exercises as focal points for discussion. Given the practical approach of the book, clients often feel enticed to keep coming back to the group and remain engaged in the process. Go to www.eatingmindfully .com for information on how to obtain a *Mindful Eating Support Group Guide*, which outlines how to run a mindful eating support group.

If you are an individual looking for a mindful eating support group to join, see www.eatingmindfully.com and look for the group listings. This is where professionals can post information about upcoming groups.

a mindful journey

As you start this journey, keep in mind an ancient story that goes like this: A Japanese master met with a professor who wanted to learn about Zen. The professor began the meeting by immediately telling the master everything he had already studied about Zen. The master listened and began to pour tea into his visitor's cup. He poured until it was full but did not stop. The professor watched the cup overflow and shouted, "It's overfull! No more will go in!" "Like this cup," the master said, "you are full of your own opinions and speculations. How can I show you Zen unless you first empty your cup?"

As this story advises, try to put aside your preconceptions, anything you already know about managing your diet. Empty your mind of traditional diet rules and ways of thinking. You may notice that there are times when your mind is drawn back to old dieting habits and expectations about how to lose weight. When this happens, remember that you will be filling up your cup with new tools as you read.

You are now prepared to tackle this workbook. Sit back and enjoy!

CHAPTER 1

what is a mindful state of mind?

The mind is everything. What you think, you become.
—Buddha

Before you dive into mindful eating, let's first talk about the word "mindfulness." It may be a new term to you. However, mindfulness—or, more specifically, mindful eating—isn't a new concept. In fact, it is centuries old and based on the Eastern concept of mindfulness, or "pure awareness." It is defined as *being present, in the moment, in a nonjudgmental way.* What does that mean? It simply means paying closer attention to your body, habits, and triggers.

Mindfulness, in general, is actually a simple concept. To put it in very basic terms, it is just about being *more aware.* You can practice mindfulness in almost everything you do. When you walk mindfully, you slow down, enjoy the scenery, and think about where you step. When you eat mindfully, you are more aware and attuned to the factors that lead you to eat even when you are full and starve yourself when you are really hungry.

The point of being mindful is to develop a close relationship with your own mind. You become familiar with what you are thinking and feeling, and less reactive to the emotions, thoughts, and cravings you have. We often act without conscious thought or awareness of why we do what we do. But when you are mindful, you accept whatever comes up in your mind or heart without judgment or criticism. You use what comes into your awareness in order to learn you more about yourself. If you are feeling sad, for example, you accept it and work through it rather than compartmentalize it or push it away. In addition, when you are mentally and physically present, you increase your enjoyment in your life. Mindfulness allows you to concentrate without distraction in the midst of all of life's white noise.

In contrast, mindlessness involves automatic, habitual thoughts and actions. It's like what Bill Murray's character experiences in the movie *Groundhog Day*: a life that is repetitive, scripted, and stuck in a rut. Contributing to this repetitive type of mindlessness is the myth about the benefits of multitasking. I recently passed a bumper sticker that read, "Multitasking Queen." It made me pause to think. The Western world takes a lot of pride in multitasking. But how much does it truly help you? Do you really get more done, or does it leave you more vulnerable to making mistakes? Similarly, consider the technological advances to cell phones, faxes, and modems just in the past ten years, which increase the pressure to multitask and put the world in fast-forward mode. Older versions of these devices seem to move at a snail's pace. You may notice how much you can't live without your cell phone or e-mail. Yet, at the same time, you feel annoyed or overwhelmed whenever you receive an e-mail or phone message. Who can keep up? The pace is mentally and physically exhausting, but slowing down seems nearly impossible.

Mealtimes don't escape this pressure. When you sit down to eat, are your thoughts stuck in fast-forward mode? Does your mind have trouble slowing down while you are sitting still at the table? Thinking and moving at a breakneck pace makes it hard to calmly and rationally think through each bite. You might rely on autopilot eating behaviors—simple, quick actions that require little thought. For example, perhaps your default mode is to eat everything on your plate. You chow down on the entire portion of meatloaf sitting on your plate rather than think through how much would be enough. You can get stuck in habits and at times even be unable to see what's happening. This is one reason why mindless eating can creep up on you. Mindless eaters are in desperate need of finding a new way of being in their bodies or a new way of understanding how they relate to food.

Here is an example of mindfulness: You are experiencing mindfulness right now as you are reading this book. As you keep your attention on the page and thoughtfully consider each word without thinking whether this is "good" or "bad," you are just reading. If you weren't mindfully reading, you'd be thinking about something else as your eyes scanned the page. You might "read" five pages and then suddenly realize you have no idea what you just read. Your hand was turning the pages, but you didn't absorb any of the content. Mindless eating is similar to mindless reading. Your hand picks up the fork, but your mind is somewhere else.

Many people around the world, from all walks of life, use and enjoy mindfulness techniques: lawyers, teachers, farmers, monks, professionals, women, and men. They practice these techniques for every reason under the sun. There are even several centers devoted to teaching children how to be mindful. Hospitals and therapists teach people mindfulness skills every day as a primary way to cope with pain and emotional suffering.

Mindful eating has caught on around the world. On the Web, you can locate numerous clinics and centers putting mindful eating into practice. These centers and doctors have helped people make mindful practices part of their everyday lives. You can find mindful eating everywhere from university counseling centers to schools, day care centers, and hospitals. The research conducted to date all points in the same direction: mindfulness interventions are

---

Mindfulness Tip: *Give Yourself a Wake-Up Call*

The next time your phone rings, use it as a reminder to focus on the moment. When you hear that ring, check in with yourself for just a second. Notice where your attention was directed in the moment before it rang. Make note of how this exercise shifts your awareness.

effective in helping people regulate their eating habits (Kristeller, Baer, and Quillian-Wolever 2006; Smith et al. 2006; Wilson 1996).

Many people have written about mindful eating over the years. In *Eat, Drink, and Be Mindful,* I take an in-depth look at the way mindfulness skills aid people in altering problematic eating and body image issues. However, *Eat, Drink, and Be Mindful* adds a unique spin on the concept. I integrate traditional mindfulness skills with cognitive behavioral techniques for eating issues. I also give real-life examples from my work with clients.

mindfulness and psychology: the benefits

Over the past few years, psychologists have begun intensively researching mindfulness. They wanted to better understand why mindfulness is therapeutic to so many people. It has been scientifically proven to help people with a vast range of emotional and physical disorders. According to research conducted over the past twenty-five years, mindfulness meditation training can do all of the following:

- Decrease depression

- Decrease anxiety

- Help a person cope with eating disorders

- Reduce fatigue and anxiety

- Improve self-esteem

- Increase tolerance to stress

- Decrease health care costs

- Decrease pain levels and the experience of pain

- Slow the heart rate and decrease blood pressure

- Strengthen the body's immune system

- Increase the ability to relax

- Improve health

(Baer 2003; Baer, Fischer, and Huss 2005a; Brown, Ryan, and Creswell 2007; Davidson et al. 2003; Kabat-Zinn 1990)

How can mindfulness provide all of these positive benefits? Paying attention to the present moment can improve the functioning of the body and brain. It does this in two specific ways.

The first way is to help you to be less reactive. When you slow down, you think more clearly. You *respond* thoughtfully instead of *reacting.* Typically, people use the same coping mechanism over and over, repeatedly reacting in the same way without thinking. Sometimes the coping mechanism is a healthy one, like going for a jog when you are frustrated. But sometimes people react by turning to substances like alcohol and drugs or food. When you slow down, you can consciously pick a new coping mechanism that is healthier. So, being mindful helps you be more aware of how you unconsciously and consciously *react* to stress and find new ways to deal with the situation without leaning on eating.

The second way is to help you relax your body. The short-term effects of mindfulness on the body are similar to the benefits of relaxation. When you are in a mindful state, you experience a measurable decrease in perspiration, slower heart rate, and changes in alpha waves in your brain. These physiological changes are evidence that your body is going into a relaxation mode. To state the obvious: your body can't be relaxed and stressed at the same time. And, when you are relaxed, you think clearer. As a result of this clarity, you tend to make wiser food decisions.

New research has suggested that mindfulness can help you both in the moment and over the long term (Davidson et al. 2003). It can change the neural connections in your brain, and it has other positive benefits. Dr. Richard Davidson, the director of the Laboratory for Affective Neuroscience at the University of Wisconsin, with his colleagues, studied the effects of mindfulness on the brain. In subjects who meditated (compared to those who didn't), they found significant increases in activity in parts of the brain that are associated with positive emotions. The same study found that the people who meditated had a significant increase in their immunity to illness.

Dr. Davidson also looked at people who had been meditating for a long time, such as monks. He found that they had created new neural pathways in their brains with long-term use of this practice. This is similar to what happens to someone who has played a sport for a very long time: with lots of repeated practice, the person's brain develops shortcuts.

For more information on how mindfulness changes your brain chemistry and way of being, you may wish to consult *The Mindful Brain: Reflection and Attunement in the Cultivation of Well-Being* by Daniel J. Siegel.

mindfulness and eating issues

Eating-disorder therapists were curious about whether mindfulness could be a helpful component of eating-disorder treatments (Kristeller and Hallett 1999; Proulx 2008; Safer et al. 2002; Smith et al. 2006; Wiser and Telch 1999). Could mindful eating really help people overcome eating problems, which are among the most difficult psychological issues out there? They found that it did!

A number of well-known therapies that have mindfulness as a main element or component are used to help people recover from eating issues. Dialectical behavior therapy (DBT), acceptance and commitment therapy (ACT), and mindfulness-based eating awareness training (MB-EAT) all use mindfulness as an important component in their treatments.

To date, researchers have found many benefits of mindfulness, as you will see in the list on the next page. We can anticipate that the interest in mindful eating is likely to grow exponentially in the next few years as more research is conducted.

how to be mindful

At this point, you may be wondering, "But how do I practice mindfulness? How do I actually do it?" Learning to be mindful is an ongoing process and takes practice. You won't master it overnight. As you read this book, you will do exercises that gradually teach you how to be mindful about managing your weight and eating habits. In the exercise below, you'll begin your mindfulness practice.

mindfulness exercise: taking a mindful moment ─────────────

Being mindful is like performing a virus scan on your computer. Sure, it takes some time now, but in the long run, those few moments will save you many hours that you would have to spend trying to recoup your computer and irreplaceable files. Running regular checks on your computer is important, because even when things appear to be running smoothly, viruses have a way of lurking in the background. Most of the time, you have no idea they are there unless you take the time to check in.

It's important to practice being mindful. It should be an activity that is done on a daily basis. It doesn't have to be a formal meditation practice; instead, you just take one minute or two to stop, reflect, and do a mini self-scan. This is simply the process of checking in with your thoughts, feelings, and sensations. So, let's take a moment to practice it.

1. Set aside a few quiet moments. Close your eyes, if that feels comfortable.

2. Focus on getting in the right frame of mind. Try to relax. Think of this task as a way to check all of your own internal files.

3. Then just ask yourself a few basic questions. Ask yourself, "How am I feeling right now? Is there anything troubling me? How does my body feel? Am I in the moment? Is there anything on my mind that is distracting me or causing me to worry? Am I smiling? Are my muscles tense?"

4. Also run through the secret or hidden files that no one else is privy to. This is the process of reflecting on deeply personal or emotional questions. Try asking yourself some of the tougher or more uncomfortable questions like "Am I feeling anxious today? Why am I feeling so stressed? Why did that statement just hurt my feelings?" If you go without doing a mindful self-scan, a lot of invisible emotions and thoughts can quietly sabotage how you function.

5. If you respond well to imagery, the next time you want to be mindful, imagine yourself hitting a button to perform an internal scan. Visualize the screen of a computer. Imagine that there are several files on the desktop. What kind of files are there? Stress? Anger? Hunger?

People often do a self-scan when things aren't working, but I encourage you to do routine maintenance on a regular basis: check in even when things are running smoothly. To help yourself become a master at doing self-scans, learn the language of mindfulness.

learning the language of mindfulness

You can start becoming a more mindful person by learning the *language* of mindfulness. Speaking mindfully means being fully aware of what you say. It also means speaking compassionately to yourself and others. Not many people know mindfulness as a first language.

Speaking mindfully takes practice. If you were taking a Spanish or French lesson, you would repeat the words over and over again in your head at first. You would repeatedly stop and work to remember the correct word until it began to come to you without having to think about it. The same happens with the language of mindfulness. When you practice thinking and talking in a language that supports compassion and awareness, over time it begins to come to you without any effort on your part.

Why should you take the time to learn this language? Language is important because words guide your actions. If you label a feeling you are having as "fear," you will run. If you identify that same feeling as "anger," you may hit something. You can see how this translates into the treatment of yourself and your body. If you describe yourself using compassionate, nonjudgmental terms, you are more likely to care for yourself. You will show your body more respect. On the contrary, imagine how you would treat yourself if you described yourself as "fatso" or "slob"; you would act in punishing and shaming ways toward your body. If you are not sure how well you know the language of mindfulness or how it fits into your life, try taking the test below.

mindfulness test

When you have trouble living mindfully, you often have difficulty eating mindfully. Here are some common ways in which people act mindlessly. Put an *X* next to the statements that apply to you.

_____ There are times when I am not really aware of what I am feeling or doing. I sometimes feel like a robot just going through the motions.

_____ I find it hard to accept myself and circumstances as they are. I often wish for something different.

_____ I sometimes make unnecessary mistakes because I'm not paying attention.

_____ I often avoid painful things, or I procrastinate so I don't have to deal with things that bother me.

_____ Sometimes I'm so consumed with my thoughts (about food or my own issues) that I'm not as social as I could be.

_____ I'm focused on just getting there. I power walk to where I am going without really noticing the scenery. Sometimes I don't even look up. I drive without really thinking about where I am going.

_____ I'm not listening very closely when other people are talking, or I find it difficult to listen to others for long periods.

_____ If I am at a lecture, half of my attention is on the speaker and the other half is somewhere else.

_____ I'm always making a mental list of what I have to do, even during inappropriate times (while I should be paying attention to work, during sex, and other times).

_____ At parties, I can't remember new people's names.

_____ I hurry through activities just to get them over with.

_____ I think I will finally be happy in the future when I have accomplished a variety of goals; I have trouble seeing what I've already done well.

_____ I sometimes drive or act on autopilot.

_____ I am bored with routine activities.

_____ I have a hard time enjoying the moment, even when I am doing something fun.

_____ I'm typically thinking, "Okay, what's next?"

_____ I dwell a lot on the past. When I start to think about painful things from the past, I can get very stuck. I have a hard time pulling myself out of it.

_____ I think a lot about the future and as a result sometimes don't enjoy what I'm doing right now.

_____ Sometimes I forget whether I've completed routine tasks because I do them so mindlessly (for example, I can't remember if I locked the door or turned off the TV when I left).

Most of us would check a few of these statements; it's a pretty normal part of day-to-day life to be mindless occasionally. However, if you marked several of these examples, you may want to commit to creating a more mindful lifestyle.

> *The most precious gift we can offer others is our presence. When mindfulness embraces those we love, they will bloom like flowers.*
> —Thich Nhat Hanh

mindfulness exercise: shifting into a mindful gear ——————

The following is a two-part exercise. First, try the activity. Then, reflect on what you learned from completing it. This will help you clarify what you experience emotionally when you shift your mind and body into a mindful gear.

Part One

Today, try to be mentally present when you are talking with someone. Perhaps it is a boss or your spouse. If you notice that your mind wanders when this person is talking to you (and it will wander!), try to bring it back to what he or she is saying. Focus on the person's facial features, tone, and expression. Notice the person's reaction to your being more present.

Part Two

Now, write down your thoughts about your experience with being more present.
Whom did you try to be more present with today?

_____

_____

What challenges did you encounter?

_____

_____

Where did your mind want to escape to? What were you thinking about? Why was it difficult to hold your focus on the discussion at hand?

_____

_____

How did this person respond when you were truly present? Did you notice a shift in body language? Perhaps a sense of appreciation? Or surprise that you were intently listening?

_____

_____

noticing mindfulness in everyday life

People use mindfulness skills every day, whether they are aware of it or not. Therapists, for example, rely heavily on mindfulness skills in their work. When a client is talking, the therapist must be present in the moment and listening very carefully. Therapists also practice nonjudgment; they try to focus on having compassion toward their clients. When clients feel that they aren't being judged, they are more likely to open up and be honest with themselves and the therapist, making it possible for them to look candidly at their behavior and make amazing changes.

Like therapists, you too already use mindfulness in your life. Write in the space below the ways in which you currently use mindfulness. Think about different roles you play. In the matter of one day, you probably wear a variety of hats: spouse, coworker, client, mother, homemaker, and others. Each of these roles brings you unique challenges, and in each of these you most likely already utilize mindfulness. List the ways you do or could use mindfulness to fulfill one of your daily roles more effectively.

_____

_____

_____

_____

_____

_____

_____

_____

_____

_____

mindful living

In this chapter, you've learned that mindfulness is a way of being in the world. It's based on awareness and being completely present. It teaches you to look at the world through open eyes, noticing rather than judging. You can use mindfulness as a way to approach anything you do in the world, in the way you work, relate to people, or deal with painful issues in your life. If you've tried it, you know that it is helpful.

As you'll discover in the following chapters, being mindful is one way to cope with eating problems, whether you are undereating or overeating. In the next chapter, you will learn how mindfulness specifically applies to changing your snacking and eating struggles.

CHAPTER 2

what is mindful eating?

Every human being is the author of his own health or disease.
—Buddha

Let's start with a brief overview of mindful eating. Mindful eating involves the development of a special kind of *awareness* that you bring to the table whenever you eat. It's not a diet. There are no rules, menus, or recipes. You don't have to cut out entire food groups like breads or meats, or count every calorie. If you've tried every diet under the sun, this probably sounds like a refreshing idea—finally, no more dieting! But, at the same time, you are probably scratching your head, wondering how this is possible.

Ronald Reagan once said, "You can tell a lot about a fellow's character by his way of eating jelly beans." Do you eat them one at a time? Savor them? Wolf them down mindlessly? Avoid them like the plague? Only in the middle of the night? In secret?

So it's true, the way you eat says a lot about you. Do you eat even when you are full? Do you continue to snack until you feel uncomfortable and bloated? Do you deprive yourself when you diet? Do you mindlessly snack on foods you don't even really like, just because they are available? Mindful eating is less about *what* you eat (healthy or junk foods) and more about the *way* you eat. Everyone knows the true secret to maintaining one's weight: only eat the amount of calories your body needs in order to function properly. It sounds simple enough. But, as you know, it's not simple at all. What stands in the way of doing what you know is best for your body? That's what this book is all about.

When you are a mindful eater, you become more aware of your eating habits, particularly those that sabotage eating well. It's like getting well acquainted with the CEO of your brain, the part in charge of making eating decisions. You learn to ask and answer questions like "Do I really want a snack?" "Am I just reacting to food with automatic habits?" "Am I mindlessly wandering to the vending machine at work and buying my favorite treat without a second thought?" Sometimes you make better decisions: you eat very mindfully. And, sometimes you don't: you eat way too much and then hate yourself for it. But you'll have more awareness of these choices, and more compassion toward yourself, even when you make unhelpful choices.

Mindful eating is not a militant program aimed at scaring you away from eating. In fact, it is quite the opposite. It lets you know that eating is okay! Eating is a good thing, and a necessary part of life.

three steps to mindful eating using the mind and mouth

There are three basic steps of mindful eating. Each of these aspects is important; combined, they allow you to be the best mindful eater you can be. Notice that the three steps direct your attention toward being keenly aware of what you are eating. But, they also stress the importance of how you think and feel about food.

1. **Tune in to the physical characteristics of food.** Pay close attention to your senses. Notice how the food tastes. Use your tongue to feel the texture. Gauge the temperature. Take a whiff of the aroma. Think of your mouth as being like a magnifying glass, zooming in. Imagine that each bite is magnified 100 percent. Ask yourself, "How does it really taste? What does it feel like in my mouth? Is this something I really want? Does it satisfy my taste buds? Is my mind truly present when I take a bite so that I experience it fully?"

2. **Tune in to repetitive habits and the process of eating.** Notice how you eat. Pay attention to when you are eating while on autopilot. In autopilot mode, you are more likely to act out of habit: eat a snack at the same time each day, multitask while you eat, or eat the same foods over and over again. Ask yourself, "Is there something I do over and over again that lends itself to mindless eating? Do I have any ingrained habits concerning how I snack? When I pick up my fork, what stands in the way of my feeling in control?"

3. **Tune in to mindless eating triggers.** Be keenly aware of what prompts you to start and stop eating. Is your kitchen a hot spot for snacking? Does a hard day (or other feelings, such as stress, discomfort, or boredom) lead to a food binge? Or, do judgmental thoughts like "I'm an idiot!" trigger mindless eating? Become an expert on the things that push you to eat when you aren't physically hungry; when you know your triggers, you can anticipate them before they happen and make better choices. Ask yourself, "What am I feeling? Am I physically or emotionally hungry? Is my environment, emotional state, or dining companion helping or hurting my efforts to eat mindfully?"

Mindful eating involves what I call the "taste patrol." Imagine the moment you spy a police car while you are cruising on a freeway. What happens the very moment you see the red and blue lights? There is this sudden shift in your attention. You check on what you are doing. "How fast am I going? How heavy is my foot on the gas pedal?" you ask yourself. You notice a sense of guilt or worry. A lot happens in that moment.

This is similar to the way you can shift your attention to your eating during a meal. Imagine that feeling you get when you see a police car, and remind yourself to check in and slow down. But don't beat yourself up!

seven skills of a mindful eater

Although mindful eating is a simple concept, it is hard to adequately put it into words, because being mindful is an experience. It's like trying to describe being head over heels in love. You can talk about it, but unless you've felt the intensity of passion firsthand, you might have a hard time understanding the experience fully. To help you understand this idea, I have broken it down into seven key skills.

The skills of mindful eating include developing *awareness,* or being more in tune with your experience. Let's take a closer look at each of the seven skills.

Awareness

Awareness is the cornerstone of mindfulness. It is calm and focused attention. In mindful eating you can focus your attention in two ways. One method is to tune in to your senses. You pay close attention to the external world: what you hear, see, touch, and, most important, taste. This method helps you notice foods you eat so frequently that you no longer pay attention to them, for example, that daily bowl of cereal that you don't really taste anymore.

To do this, closely track the sensations in your body: hunger, stress, pain, and emotions. This is harder than it sounds. These sensations help you to really taste food and know when it is time to stop eating. But really, how often do you take a moment to think about the basic sensations of eating? Experiences are often taken as a whole without breaking them down into parts.

Many of my clients talk about misreading their body. They always feel hungry. Or, they eat until they feel too full. It's no surprise that this is such a difficult skill. Years of mindlessly overeating and dieting can warp the way you hear and respond to your body's signals. When you are really aware of what's going on inside, you hear the very subtle internal feedback your body gives you. You can use this information as a guide to deciding when to stop and start eating.

The second method of awareness has to do with getting to know the habits that hang you up. A habit is like a groove in a worn-out tire: it makes you veer a certain way. Maybe, for example, you have a habit of munching on food while standing up over the sink. Or, you might wander into the kitchen each time you need to wind down from your day. These habits veer you toward mindless eating and become pitfalls in the mindful eating process. As you read this book, don't be surprised if you begin to notice habits and thoughts about yourself that weren't on your radar screen before. Once you are aware of them, you can start to develop different habits.

Observation

When you observe, you see a situation from a distance, like watching yourself on a movie screen. It's so much easier to see the entire story line when you are watching the movie rather than participating as an actor in the middle of it. And, because you are just observing, you don't try to change the experience or deal with it. You just notice, as if you are an impartial witness. So, when a thought about food pops into your head, the impartial witness inside you gives a gentle nudge and says, "Did you notice that? A thought about food just popped into your head again."

When you closely observe your body, feelings, and thoughts, you start to understand the tricky feelings and subtle situations that trigger mindless eating. You learn to observe your body's hints that tell you when you are full or hungry. Observing your thoughts is a little trickier. Many people get caught up in what they are thinking. A more important skill is to know why you are thinking about snacking at that very moment, and what type of thought it is. What prompted this thought? How does the thought affect your actions?

Being in the Moment

When you don't even have to think about how to do something, like driving a car or walking, it becomes automatic, freeing your mind to think about past mistakes or future worries. The same is true of eating. Eating, like brushing your teeth or driving a car, doesn't require much conscious thought. For this reason, you are often not really mentally present at the table. This lack of presence may be linked to one of the many underlying causes of mindless eating. When we are not consciously thinking about our food consumption, we can very easily develop unhealthy habits around eating, eating too much at restaurants or digging unconsciously into the snack drawer at our desk. Mindful eating helps you act consciously instead of out of habit.

Where is your mind when it's not in the immediate moment? It can be so many places! Your thoughts may dwell on the past. Have you ever run a red light because you were beating yourself up over a recent mistake you had made? Or, you may be obsessing about the future. However, when you are in the moment, your mind notices things *as they happen*. Making sure your mind sits with you at the table helps you make mindful decisions about what to eat.

Being Mindful of the Environment

Notice how your environment encourages or discourages you from acting in a mindful way. People are very hard on themselves for mindless eating, but who could blame them when they are constantly inundated with TV commercials for junk food, and restaurants serve portions that are big enough to feed three people?

When you pay attention to your environment, you notice how many things around you trigger mindless eating. In addition to noticing commercials and ads that encourage mindless overeating, also notice ads that try to sabotage your appetite. Advertisements for diets and images of stick-thin, airbrushed fashion models can lead to unrealistic expectations of yourself, often turning on the urge to starve yourself.

While reading this book, you'll be working on noticing what's around you and making your environment more mindful. Do you own a lot of diet books? Are there people around you who are frequently talking about diets or obsessing about their weight? Do you stock your kitchen with healthy or junk food? Take inventory of the mindless eating environment around you.

Nonjudgment

It's easy to criticize and scrutinize every bite. People can be so hard on themselves, particularly over the way they eat. Instead of supporting judgmental thoughts, mindfulness trains people to think neutrally or compassionately. In other words, things don't always have to be labeled as "good" or "bad." Things are what they are. You can learn to be empathetic about the difficulty of mindful eating. As you stop judging, you allow yourself to be more present and aware of what you are doing.

It's not as if you can magically make judgments go away. When they are present, you just notice judgments like "I am such an idiot. I just blew it," without necessarily believing the judgmental and critical thoughts. Even though people often try to use guilt and name calling to try to motivate change, compassion and empathy are what actually help people move forward.

Letting Go

Freedom from eating problems and peace of mind come when you stop holding on to the way you think things "should be": fitting into a certain pants size, eating in a particular way, having it all together. Instead, when you let go, you allow the situation to be as it is without wishing for something better. Sometimes it means giving something up that you really wanted and maybe believed you couldn't live without. For many clients, this has meant giving up the dream of being a size two.

A continual struggle is around letting go of food cravings. When a food craving hits, many people are at a total loss regarding how to answer it wisely. An even bigger challenge is to let go of the desire to be in complete in control, the wish to be the kind of person who eats perfectly and never slips up. And letting go of being in control is a lot harder than it sounds.

When you get the hang of letting go, this allows you to let strong feelings pass by without acting on them. Psychologists often use the phrase "Feel the feelings." What does that mean? It means feeling painful emotions without running to something (food or alcohol) to numb the feeling. The emotions are often more tolerable than you think. In fact, learning to identify and cope with feelings is sometimes more important than throwing out the junk food and eating fruits and vegetables, since it's possible to mindlessly overeat healthy food when you're running from difficult feelings.

Acceptance

Acceptance means being okay with the way things are. You don't have to like it or agree with the situation, but you acknowledge and work with the situation as it is. Too often, people fight so hard against having the problem that they never get around to taking steps to do something about it. They get stuck in stewing about the unfairness. As the saying goes, "Acceptance is the first step in dealing with any problem." From there, you can move on.

Acceptance can also help you heal a damaged body image. You learn how to say "I am who I am" without trying to change. This is extremely tough for many people. Eventually, people come to realize that acceptance is a little like the way you feel about your shoe size. You might think that your feet are too big or too small, but you've learned to work with the situation as it is. You can't do much to change the size of your foot, but you do work on taking good care of your feet, and sometimes you might dress up your feet in nice shoes.

Not accepting yourself is damaging emotionally and physically. You can easily get caught in punishing yourself by depriving yourself of food or wearing uncomfortable clothes, or you might rob yourself of good times, avoiding hanging out with friends because you are afraid to be in a bathing suit around them.

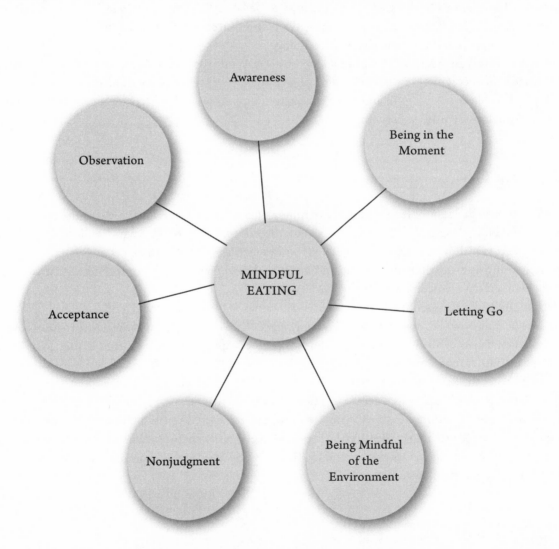

Each of the above is a separate skill. When used together they create the experience of mindfulness. It's like swimming: to swim, you combine a variety of individual skills: special breathing, kicking, moving your arms, and treading water. Once you get the hang of swimming, you do it automatically without thought. But if you've never been swimming before, you have to draw your attention to each action. You practice your breathing technique or arm strokes. With eating mindfully, as with swimming, if you don't get the hang of using these skills right away, you can develop them over time with practice.

Some of these skills may be very easy for you. You may have developed them in other places in your life. For example, if someone close to you has died suddenly, it's likely that you've already had to work on acceptance. You know the suffering and agony that goes along with hating the way things are; the desire for things to be different can drive you crazy when it is something that you can't change. Or, if you've been through an unwanted breakup, you have firsthand knowledge of the excruciating pain of trying to let go when you don't want to. Other skills may be quite difficult for you to learn. Let's take a look at Cindy's experience to see how these skills can be used to change mindless eating.

Putting the Seven Skills into Action

Cindy, a fifty-year-old mother of three girls and successful business manager, joined one of my mindful eating support groups because she struggled with a mild case of mindless eating that grew into a big problem. She described herself as a "hit or miss" eater. Sometimes she ate nutritious foods and reasonable portions. Other times, she had some big misses: a carton of ice cream, a plate of Christmas cookies, two bagels instead of one.

After the birth of each child, Cindy had put on weight. She had tried to take off the baby weight with a menagerie of fad diets. In her forties, she gave up trying. The pound she gained each year was difficult to hide on her petite five-foot-three-inch frame. Cindy described her closet as being like a dress shop: it contained clothes of all sizes. Her doctor, concerned about Cindy's health, would lecture her about losing weight but didn't offer any useful tips about how to do it. She always left the doctor's office frustrated and angry.

Out of desperation, she came to the mindful eating support group. Initially, she was skeptical. Managing her weight seemed like it should be a simple enough task. Cindy was a smart woman; at work, she could make a plan and execute it with no problem. So, why couldn't she do this simple task of losing weight? This illogical situation irritated her. For many people like Cindy, this is a common dilemma: if I want it, why can't I just do it?

Cindy's first challenge was to grasp the concept of letting go, the ability to stop doing things that just don't work even though you think they should. This meant letting go of the dieting mind-set, which told her that she had to starve herself and adhere to a bland regimen of oatmeal and plain salad. Like many dieters, if she told herself no more carbohydrates, she would begin to obsess about bread and pasta. In the support group, Cindy learned that she could still eat the pasta and meatballs she loved, but she had to eat them in a very different way than she had in the past.

First, she worked on moving past the idea that managing her weight was impossible. From the start, the other members of the group could tell that she didn't believe she could change her eating habits. And, of course, if she didn't believe she could do it, nothing would ever change.

Another important step toward becoming a mindful eater was mastering the art of awareness. Cindy could hardly believe that she wasn't supposed to make changes to her diet at first. Her only job was to observe her everyday behavior as it was. And for the first time, she began to notice habits that repeatedly led to mindless eating. Observing herself was shocking! Each day Cindy walked blindly into the very same mindless eating traps. For example, she ate while standing in front of the refrigerator, and she grabbed food directly from boxes in her pantry. When Cindy skimped on lunch, she snacked voraciously the moment she returned home from work. These two habits were fairly easy to fix. Cindy made a conscious effort to sit down whenever she ate and to bring a snack to work.

But Cindy had two other mindless habits that were much tougher to alter. She snacked at night when her husband worked the late shift. She found herself bored and restless at home. The leftovers from dinner in the refrigerator seemed to call her name. It was a struggle to find things to keep her occupied in the evenings when she was home alone. Also, she went out to lunch with friends two or three times a week, a huge mindless eating trap.

Cindy discovered that one or two changes can make a monumental difference. Dieting was never going get to the root of the problem. Instead, she used the seven skills to change her relationship to food. In a nutshell, Cindy stopped multitasking while she ate. She made sure every bite was a mindful bites, really tasting food. Cindy also found a new hobby, knitting, to keep her busy at night. This seemed to keep her hands occupied, and the time flew by on evenings when her husband was gone. She also discovered ways to connect with friends besides going out to dinner, such as going to a movie or out for a walk. Most important, she stopped beating herself up about her food failures in the past. This helped her to move forward.

Just focusing on changing her habits turned her life around. She didn't drastically change her diet, just her lifestyle and coping mechanisms. Not only did she stop gaining weight, which was her main goal, but she even lost weight. It happened not overnight but progressively. Soon, she actually wanted to go back to the doctor to show him the progress she had finally made.

mindfulness exercise: Do You Have the Seven Skills?

The worksheet below is a brief self-assessment of your mindless and mindful eating habits. This is not a diagnostic tool or instrument; it won't provide you with a clinical label or diagnosis. Instead, it will help you pinpoint your strengths and behaviors that could use some attention. Put a check mark by each statement that applies to you. When you're done, you may wish to focus first on the skill section with the most check marks.

Awareness

_____ I often zone out during the process of eating. I graze on food.

_____ I often eat more than I wanted to or just don't listen to what my body needs.

_____ I sometimes ignore my physical hunger; I tell myself I'm not hungry when I am.

_____ I often don't pay attention to the taste of food.

_____ I often don't notice how food smells.

_____ Sometimes I am not aware of how much I have eaten until after I'm finished.

_____ When I diet, I am anxiously focused on calories or what I eat.

_____ At times, I get stuck in my concern about some aspects of eating (fat grams, scales, weight, or sizes).

_____ I have some routines or habits regarding the way I eat.

_____ I have trouble noticing how I feel about food until after the fact, and then I feel guilty.

_____ I try to ignore my hunger until I am famished, or I try to skip meals.

Observation

_____ I often don't see what is behind my mindless eating; I just do it without analyzing it.

_____ I sometimes don't see how I create my own pain as I am mindlessly eating.

_____ I am not able to perceive my thoughts and feelings about food without acting on them (the moment I notice I have a craving, I have to act on it and can't let it go by).

_____ I don't listen when my body says stop.

_____ I have extreme reactions to hunger: I ignore it or obsess about it and have trouble finding a middle ground.

_____ I feel uncomfortable if I eat mindlessly and then can't exercise or compensate for it in some way.

_____ I am not aware of changes in my body, or I obsess about every detail.

_____ I have experienced coldness, dry skin, weakness, fatigue, or high blood pressure because of my eating habits or weight.

_____ I feel heavy.

_____ It's sometimes hard to find things I like to wear or feel comfortable wearing.

_____ I have a lot of physical problems, particularly due to my weight.

_____ I often feel fat or anxious about the shape or size of my body.

Being in the Moment

_____ I sometimes obsess about what my body looked like in the past or could look like in the future rather than accept who I am now.

_____ When I notice my mind wandering while I'm eating, it's hard to bring myself back into the present moment.

_____ I often eat little handfuls of food without thinking about it.

_____ My thoughts about food often tend to run away from me.

_____ I often multitask when I eat.

_____ I often eat while standing up.

_____ I often eat in front of the TV.

_____ My mind is a whirl of thoughts. It's hard to focus just on eating because I have so much on my mind.

_____ I'm so busy that it's hard to find time to focus on what I eat.

_____ I'm drawn to foods that are convenient to prepare, such as snacks or microwavable foods.

_____ Making dinner seems like a chore; it's hard to enjoy the process.

_____ Sometimes eating seems to take up a lot of my time and energy that could be focused on other things.

Being Mindful of the Environment

_____ I have a lot of food that I eat mindlessly in a handy, convenient place (in my kitchen or on my desk).

_____ I read a lot of fashion magazines that have articles about dieting.

_____ I own a candy dish or cookie jar.

_____ I eat at a lot of fast-food restaurants.

_____ I watch TV shows that prompt me to feel bad about my body.

_____ I watch a lot of TV.

_____ I go for a lot of convenient foods (like snack foods and foods that are easy to microwave).

_____ I feel as if I don't have time to eat.

_____ My friends are mindless eaters.

_____ My culture focuses a lot on eating.

_____ The majority of my extended family members have struggled with mindless eating.

_____ I have friends who are competitive about their weight.

_____ I talk a lot about dieting.

_____ I notice billboards and advertisements for food.

_____ I find myself having cravings when I see pictures of good food on magazine covers or on TV.

_____ I like a bargain and find that I buy things in bulk despite the fact that the quantity is too much food for my household.

_____ I watch TV programs about preparing food.

Letting Go

_____ I crave or cling to the idea of losing weight. I can't let it go. It's on my mind a lot and clouds my judgment at times.

_____ When I have the urge to eat, I have to act on it, even if I'm not really hungry.

_____ I can't seem to move past the idea that dieting is the answer.

_____ I think about food often, even when I should be focusing on other things.

_____ I think obsessively about my body and food.

_____ I often can't just let things go; I ruminate about them for a long time.

_____ It doesn't seem like my thoughts about food come and go; they seem to linger.

_____ I worry about letting go of my current habits, because I am afraid of failing.

Nonjudgment

_____ I get mad at myself for worrying about eating so much.

_____ I label myself as bad when I mindlessly eat.

_____ I don't like to eat with other people because they may judge me or my body.

_____ I eat mindlessly when I'm emotional.

_____ I get mad at myself when I eat mindlessly or feel that I've messed up.

_____ I avoid eating sometimes when I feel bad, as a way of punishing myself.

_____ My relationships have been affected by my eating habits (I don't feel self-confident; I have avoided an intimate moment with a loved one due to feeling fat; I have avoided a relationship; I've wanted to be thinner than friends).

_____ I feel fat and often label myself with this word.

_____ Guilt rules my decisions about what to eat or not eat.

_____ I get competitive or jealous of other people's bodies.

_____ I think critical thoughts about myself and my body.

_____ My thoughts are often judgmental.

Acceptance

_____ I often wish for a different body.

_____ It's hard for me to appreciate the good things about my body; I don't believe there are any good features to my body.

_____ I find eating to be a hard or unpleasant experience.

_____ It makes me very mad that I have to deal with eating issues.

_____ I am often jealous of other people who don't struggle with their weight.

_____ I often think that I don't want this to be a problem or that it "shouldn't" be a problem.

_____ I feel like a failure because I can't get it right.

_____ I have trouble accepting my body as it is.

_____ I have difficulty appreciating things I do like about my body; I ignore the positives and focus on the negatives.

Use the space below to write about the area of mindful eating that is the most challenging to you. What did you learn from this exercise? Use this information to determine which skill needs extra attention. If you find yourself having trouble being in the moment, for example, be sure to focus more attention to that section of the book.

_____

_____

_____

_____

when are you cured?

How will you know when you have successfully conquered mindless eating? Perhaps you're thinking, "I'll know I'm through with mindless overeating when my craving for pumpkin pie is gone or I stop wanting to gobble up cheese-covered fries." Wrong! These urges to eat the foods you love may never go away. They're normal. These foods taste great and entice everyone's taste buds.

If you are a mindful eater, you accept the hard reality of that urge to eat cheesecake and chocolate chip cookies. You just respond to that urge in a different way. A mindless eater responds to, or acts on, almost every urge. A mindful eater acts on some of these desires to eat yummy foods. The good news is that, once you start to respond mindfully to urges to eat, you will notice a change in your desire for food. The urges won't be so scary anymore, and the longing for food won't be as strong over time.

Mindless Eating and Undereating

Mindful eating is ideal for overeaters. They calm their turbulent relationship with food, the primary problem most mindless eaters face. Slowing down and connecting to the process of eating and noticing their body's cues helps mindless eaters make wiser food choices.

Mindful eating is also ideal for chronic undereaters, yo-yo dieters, and people who restrict their food in unhealthy ways. I use many of these worksheets with clients who are dealing with serious eating concerns like anorexia and bulimia, in conjunction with therapy and other forms of medical treatment.

If you've ever had a chronic problem with eating, you know that disordered eating is not really about food or appearance. Although popular magazines give the perception that the pursuit of thinness or an ideal body image fuels anorexia and chronic dieting, the problem is much deeper and more complex. It is less about appearance and more about lack of self-worth, shame, difficulty tolerating emotions, a need for control, and problems with self-acceptance. That is why telling someone with an eating problem to "just eat" doesn't even scratch the surface. It's more about helping the person learn to feel anxiety and discomfort without pushing the pain away through starvation and binging or purging. When you are able to be mindful of painful feelings without reacting to them by turning to (or away from) food, you've got the hang of it.

Mindful eating doesn't happen overnight. But working with a trained therapist using this approach can help you reorganize the grip that eating issues have over you. There are some key reasons why mindful eating is helpful in straightening out these core issues.

I recently treated a woman, Cecily, who had been struggling with yo-yo dieting and restricting for five years. She is a good example of an undereater who used mindful eating to recover. She had been restricting calories and yo-yo dieting for a long time. She was tired, irritable, and scared of most foods. However, she was determined to be healthier again.

When she entered therapy, her first words were, "Just tell me what to eat." After years of ignoring her hunger, she didn't know when she was full or hungry. She began by taking mindful bites, paying attention to nutrition, and observing patterns she had developed around food. Stress and the feeling that she was not good enough had driven her to extreme dieting. When she was on the road to recovery, she was able to identify those feelings and use non-food-coping mechanisms to deal with the feelings rather than restricting. She now uses mindful eating on a daily basis.

In this book, you will see how the exercises are great for everyone, whether you have a problem with overeating, undereating, or chronic dieting.

The Starving Mind

If you are significantly underweight or have other chronic mental health issues like untreated depression, you might need medical intervention before mindful eating is helpful to you. It's important to meet with medical and mental health professionals who can help you get to a healthy state of mind. When your body is deep in starvation mode, it's difficult to be truly mindful and present. Your mind becomes clouded by obsessive thoughts of food.

Starvation studies conducted by Ancel Keys during World War II at the University of Minnesota prove this fact. In this landmark study, researchers, knowing that people were starving in Europe due to the war, wanted to establish the best way of refeeding these people once the war was over. This study found that starvation and even semi-starvation kicks the body into a particularly difficult mode. The body attempts to defend against the lack of food by triggering hunger, a cognitive state that motivates people to eat; but people also begin to obsess about food in unhealthy ways. Most of what we know about the cognitive and emotional impact of starvation comes from the Keys study (Kalm and Semba 2005). The study was conducted with a group of healthy American men who had been screened for mental and physical problems. The goal was to track the effects of a twenty-four-week period of semi-starvation. During the study, a few subjects dropped out, and the others developed habits they had never had before, like binge eating, stealing food, severe depression, and symptoms of psychosis. The researchers were surprised that men who had never previously obsessed or worried about food had such severe symptoms. Over fifty years later, a follow-up study was done. They found men from the study and interviewed them about their current eating behavior. All of the men still worried about what they ate or reported having problematic habits around food.

If you've ever dieted, your body has probably gotten a glimpse of the effect of semi-starvation. Dieters are the first to tell you that they notice a huge increase in thinking about food when they diet, but not in a positive way. Their cravings get out of control. This is because they are ignoring their body's natural cue to eat. It's like turning off the ringer on your phone when someone is really trying to contact you. It's likely that the person will eventually find a way to track you down that you can't ignore. If you want to be mindful, you have to feed your brain; you can't starve it. An adequately fed mind has an easier time being mindful.

the mindful eating motto

I chose the title of this book purposefully, playing off the popular saying "Eat, drink, and be merry." What does the phrase bring to mind? It probably conjures up an image of people feasting happily at a party without a care in the world. It also gives the message that you need food to enjoy yourself. If you've picked up this book, you have probably experienced many times when food was not full of merriment; most likely quite the opposite. You know that you can't lean on food to make you happy. This is a recipe for disaster. You can, however, use your experiences with food to help you be more mindful.

So, "Eat, drink, and be mindful" is the motto of this book, and I hope it will become your motto too.

Make "Eat, drink, and be mindful" your mantra.

A mantra is any phrase or sound that you repeat to yourself frequently. The words have the power to change the direction of your thoughts. You may not realize that you unconsciously repeat many unhealthy mantras to yourself all the time. For example, sayings like "I'll start my diet on Monday" and "Oh well, I blew it anyway" are dieting mantras. Say "Eat, drink, and be mindful" to yourself over and over again. Call this phrase to mind whenever you are struggling with a food choice or need to get back on track. If you repeat it enough, you will begin to notice yourself saying, when you make a healthy food decision, "Wow, I am eating, drinking, and being mindful."

---

mindful eating 101

In this chapter, you learned the basic elements of mindful eating and the mindful eating motto. To sum up, it's okay to enjoy eating. Eating is fun. It also serves a very specific purpose: to provide nourishment, energy, and pleasure, and be a source of life. The trick is to eat wholesome foods with a mindful spirit.

You will continue to gain practice and knowledge about how to put the seven skills into use. Keep the mindful eating motto, "Eat, drink, and be mindful," on your mind. Use it as a simple, daily reminder to stay mindful during meals.

In the next chapter, you will begin to take a much closer look at your current eating habits through a number of self-assessments.

CHAPTER 3

a mindful eating self-assessment

Now that you have learned the basics of mindful eating, it's time to take a closer look at your day-to-day eating patterns. Perhaps you've wondered how to know if you are a mindful or mindless eater. Maybe you've compared yourself to a close family member or a friend. When you've put your eating habits side by side with your sister's diet, you seem to be doing pretty well. You eat well-rounded meals and occasionally wrestle with mindless eating in the presence of bacon and Italian food. However, when measured against a coworker's lunch, your portion sizes are much bigger, and this makes you think you may be overeating. Or, perhaps you eat a well-balanced diet on most days but struggle with mindless eating during the winter holiday season. Does this make you a mindless eater?

This chapter contains mini self-assessments to help you answer these questions. There is nothing tricky or complicated in the self-assessments. Just be honest with yourself, and you will find the answers that are the key to turning around your mindless eating.

getting started

When you start doing the assessments, first try to stop comparing yourself to others. Be mindful of your own habits, and keep your eyes on your own plate, so to speak. It's very difficult to compare yourself to others and get accurate information. In fact, comparing your eating habits to others' often moves you into a judgmental mode, in which you think things like "My habits are better than John's" or "My habits are worse than Mary's."

Once you have filled out the assessments to determine if you have the tendencies of a mindful or mindless eater, you will determine how ready you are to take the next step in the mindful eating journey. Are you still gathering information, or are you ready to dive in? This is extremely important. If you are still not ready to take action but start to make changes, it's likely you will set yourself up for frustration and setbacks. You probably already know what this is like; a setback can be devastating. You want to do everything possible to ensure your success.

As you do the self-assessments, you may find yourself tempted to judge where you are. You may find yourself saying, "I should have done more," "I should know better," or "I should have gotten farther than this!" If you notice yourself judging your current status, just take note of this strong pull, and instead think of these self-assessments as a tool rather than a reason for judgment. They are simply meant to focus your attention, as if shining a flashlight in a dark corner, so you can see where to place your attention.

are you a mindful eater?

The following are characteristics of mindful eaters, mindless dieters, mindless overeaters, undereaters, and chaotic eaters. This list contains a variety of key symptoms, but it is not an exhaustive list. People's mindless eating habits are expressed in many unique ways. Use this as a rough guide to see what types of mindless eating you experience. Put a check mark next to behaviors that describe yours.

Mindful Eater

_____ Flexible about eating (sweets and healthy foods in moderation)

_____ Aware of nutritional needs, able to meet body's needs

_____ Familiar and in touch with body (hunger cues, fullness)

_____ Trusts body to give accurate cues of hunger and fullness; hunger doesn't cause a lot of anxiety

_____ Comfortably eats when hungry and stops when full

_____ Nonjudgmental of self; accepting of body; notices self-criticism and can redirect thoughts

_____ Focuses on the impact of food on health and general well-being

_____ Enjoys food; doesn't get bogged down by guilt

_____ Eats mindlessly occasionally (such as on holidays or around a favorite food)

_____ Recovers quickly from any incidents of mindless eating

Mindless Dieter

_____ Has tried many different kinds of fad and yo-yo diets that don't last long

_____ Buys lots of diet products, magazines with diet tips, diet guides

_____ Feels guilty when eating something "bad" or off the diet

_____ Ignores the taste of diet food

_____ Has a body image ideal in mind and feels unhappy with self without it

_____ Scrutinizes food labels and follows "food rules"

Mindless Overeater

_____ Has ups and downs in weight

_____ Eats until feels uncomfortable; is aware of fullness but keeps eating

_____ Picks at food mindlessly; grazes on food

_____ Feels out of control and unable to stop

_____ Has intense food cravings

_____ Feels embarrassed to eat with others

_____ Uses food to comfort self or to maintain pleasant feelings

Mindless Undereater

_____ Skimps on nutritional needs

_____ Cuts out certain foods or food groups

_____ Is obsessive about calories, fat, or some other single aspect of food

_____ Worries a lot about weight

_____ Desires perfection

_____ Feels good about self when hungry

_____ Isolates instead of eating with others

_____ Fears losing control

Mindless Chaotic Eater

_____ Looks for a way to compensate for overeating (by exercising or purging)

_____ Has ups and downs in weight

_____ Sometimes purchases large amounts of food and sometimes restricts food (or has a *perceived* binge: eats a quantity of food that he or she believes is a lot but may not actually be that much)

_____ Thinks critically about self; other areas of life also seem out of control

_____ Has difficulty coping with stress; often uses food to help cope

_____ Often uses food to numb out

_____ Has many of the symptoms of overeating

_____ Feels empty

_____ Eats while doing something else and seldom feels full

This worksheet should give you a general idea of where you fall on the spectrum between mindless and mindful eating. Keep in mind that people experience eating issues in so many different ways. Some elements may be familiar to you and some may not.

---

are you ready for mindful eating?

Okay, so you've made the decision to eat more mindfully. That's great. Now what? Although you wish it would, change doesn't magically happen overnight. Instead, change is a process—a long process. It's hard to be patient. The good news is that change takes place in predictable steps. The book *Changing for Good* (Prochaska, Norcross, and DiClemente 1994) discusses the authors' extensive research into the way people make healthy changes to their behavior. Most of the behaviors people want to adopt, such as stopping smoking or increasing their exercise, can be applied to this model, which includes six essential steps.

The following chart shows how the stages would look if they were adapted to the challenges of mindful eating. Like any issue, becoming a mindful eater is a process.

STAGES OF MINDFUL EATING

Stage One: I Don't Have A Problem. I don't think I need to change my mindless eating, but other people (doctor or family) tell me I should.

Stage Two: I Have An Issue, But I'm Not Quite Ready. I am thinking about changing my mindless eating habits, but I'm not quite ready. (I want to eat more mindfully.)

Stage Three: I'm Getting Ready. I am thinking about changing and have taken some steps to get ready to work on my mindless eating. (I am reading a book, or I'm going to a counselor.)

Stage Four: I'm Changing. I am adapting my eating habits. (I am eating more appropriate portion sizes; I am eating healthier foods; I savor food and eat it slowly.)

Stage Five: I've Changed For Good. I have changed my ways. Eating mindfully doesn't take much effort. (I'm committed to eating mindfully.)

Stage Six: I've Slipped Up. Some of my old behaviors have come back and I am working on getting back on track. (I commit to eating mindfully each day.)

The stages of mindful eating are adapted from the stages of change model in *Changing for Good* (Prochaska, Norcross, and DiClemente 1994).

Think about how much more effective your efforts will be when you allow yourself to go through these stages. Instead of feeling guilty when you slip up, briefly going back to your old ways is an acceptable and normal part of the process.

I often see clients who are frustrated and angry with their doctors or mental health professionals. I believe this is frequently the result of a gap in communication or knowledge about the process of change. For example, imagine that you go to see your doctor. You are at stage two, just thinking about changing your mindless eating but not quite ready to make the changes. Your doctor wants you to skip ahead and move directly into action mode and gives you many instructions, which you aren't quite prepared or ready to follow. You feel overwhelmed because you aren't ready to put the advice into practice. You are simply in an early part of the cycle, but you end up feeling that you are not succeeding. What would be more helpful is to find interventions that are appropriate and realistic for the stage of change you are in.

In the text below, you'll find examples of the six stages, meant to help you understand the subtle distinctions between the stages. They also show you what to do next depending on the stage you are currently in. Take a moment to look at the stages, and find which one best describes you at this moment.

Stage One

"I don't think I eat mindlessly, but other people think I do."

"Are you going to eat that?" It's a phrase you've heard a lot from your friends and family lately. Sometimes they subtly hint that they are concerned about your eating habits ("Have you tried the salad here? It's great").

Other times they aren't so tactful. They flat out tell you, "Look you've got a problem. You eat way too much!" or "Your weight is an issue." Perhaps your doctor has lectured you or has advised you to change your eating habits for the sake of your health.

If you don't think you have a problem with mindless eating, but your partner, friends, or family members often nag you about your eating habits, you might fall into this category. The foods you choose to eat (or not eat) seem to bother other people in a way that doesn't concern you at the moment. Other people say things like:

- "When you stop and start dieting, it drives me crazy. I'm sick of it."

- "I'm really upset when you overeat."

- "You are not at a healthy weight."

- "You need to eat more healthy foods. You eat junk!"

- "I'm concerned about your health. You are at risk for type 2 diabetes, high blood pressure, cancer, fertility problems, and a shortened life."

Where to Focus in This Workbook

If you are not sure whether you are a mindless eater (or have an issue with food), that's okay. Perhaps someone gave you this book, or maybe you picked it up to humor your partner or you are trying to get your parents off your back. Why not try completing the mindfulness self-assessments? After you complete these worksheets, bring them back to your doctor or discuss your answers with the individual who raised the concern. You might find it beneficial to just flip through the pages to see if any of the exercises apply to you. If so, you may want to consider continuing to read further.

Stage Two

"I realize I eat mindlessly, but I'm not quite ready to change my behavior."

You have said things like:

- "I have too much going on in my life to eat mindfully."

- "It seems like a lot of effort and work."

- "I need more information on eating healthy foods."

- "I'll start on my diet after the holidays (or other events)."

- (For undereaters and dieters) "I am afraid to change my eating despite knowing it is extreme, because I'm afraid of getting fat."

- "I don't have time; I'm too stressed."

- "I've tried and feel as if I've failed in the past."

Where to Focus in This Workbook

If you are not quite ready, that is okay. You might want to start by just noticing your eating patterns. At this point, focus on the worksheets that help you specifically pinpoint the problem. Also, just read through the book. Bring it back out and start completing the exercises when you feel you are ready. Commit to reading the introduction of this book. It will give you the background information you will need when you are ready to start.

Stage Three

"I realize I eat mindlessly, and I'm getting ready to eat more mindfully."

You say things like:

- "I'm going to begin eating better on Monday."

- "I'm committed to improving my diet but fear it will be difficult."

- "I've already made a few changes, like cutting down on the junk and eating more fruits and vegetables."

- "I've started reading books on healthy eating."

- "I've looked in the phone book for some therapist referrals."

- "I'm more aware of the times I'm falling into mindless eating behavior (such as mindless snacking, engaging in emotional eating, and purging)."

- "I've begun planning a time to start."

Where to Focus in This Workbook

You are getting close to taking action. It's likely that you already know what the problem is and are anxious to make changes. Begin by doing a self-assessment. However, before you make any changes, gather as much information as possible about your habits. You might want to start with keeping a mindfulness food diary. When you complete it, don't make any changes; just try to observe. Also, it might be helpful to start working on mindful bites, slowing down when you're eating so you can focus on the taste and texture. In addition, make a contract with yourself about what you plan to do in the future to explore your mindless eating history.

You are almost ready to dive in! It's likely that you've already completed the introduction of this workbook and are ready to do the worksheets. You are working specifically on getting to know your body again. If you have found particular worksheets in this book to be useful, it's important to post them in an easily visible location in your home. These can serve as daily reminders to check in with yourself and assess your status.

Stage Four

"I'm making great changes. I am eating mindfully on a regular basis."

You say things like:

- "Now I've got the idea. I'm able to keep it going. I am even enjoying eating in a more mindful way."

- "My eating habits have really improved. I'm eating more mindfully on a daily basis."

- "When I snack, I ask myself if I'm eating mindfully.

- "I'm keeping a mindful food journal."

- "I've consulted with people who help me eat more mindfully; my partner is on board, or I've consulted with a professional (such as a nutritionist, psychiatrist, physician, or therapist)."

- "I continue to praise myself and recognize when I eat mindfully."

- "If I do eat mindlessly, I take a step back and figure out why and how to avoid it in the future."

Where to Focus in This Workbook

You've got the hang of it and have made some big changes. Of course, it is important for you to know what can trigger a relapse. It's likely that you are going to struggle the most to make mindful choices when you are in stressful situations. Make sure you complete the "Mindless Eating Relapse Prevention" worksheet in chapter 11.

Stage Five

"I eat mindfully now! I've changed my behavior."

If you have reached this stage in your journey, kudos! I take my hat off to you and applaud you. The majority of people who embark on this journey are just ecstatic to reach the fifth stage. You say things like:

- "Eating isn't a challenge for me any longer."

- "When I'm around foods that I used to mindlessly eat, they don't tempt me."

- "I don't worry about relapsing; I know I can handle it."

- "As an undereater or dieter, I no longer stress or worry about calories or what I weigh."

Where to Focus in This Workbook

Keep up the good work. Put this workbook in a handy place. Bring it out when you experience any recurrences of mindless eating. Also, share it with friends and family who are looking for help with their mindless eating.

Stage Six

"I've been eating mindfully for a long period of time.
But I've slipped up and I am eating mindlessly again."

It's bound to happen. Even the most mindful eaters should expect to slip up now and again. This doesn't mean you've failed. It shouldn't derail you. In fact, this stage is here because you should expect some challenges. This forces you to be mindful of the problem again and renew your commitment to eating mindfully. This is a continual journey!

You say things like:

- "I can't believe this happened. I was doing so well."

- "Eating mindfully had not been a problem for a long time."

- "I need to renew my commitment to eating mindfully every single day. Just because I've made some changes doesn't mean my old ways don't look tempting."

- "When I lapse back into my mindless eating, I have to be compassionate toward myself rather than hard on myself."

- "I have to get back on track. I know I can do it because I've done it in the past."

Where to Focus in This Workbook

You had mindless eating down pat. However, some of your old ways crept back. It is a normal part of the cycle to experience a brief reoccurrence of symptoms during stressful times. It is important for you to know what can trigger a relapse. It's likely that you are going to struggle the most to make mindful choices when you are in stressful situations. Make sure you complete the worksheet titled "Mindless Eating Relapse Prevention" in chapter 11. If you do have a relapse, remember to be compassionate with yourself. Get yourself back on track by determining what factors led to the slipup.

are you ready for mindful eating?

It's likely that you've been at each of the six stages at several times in your life. Answer the insight questions below to understand what causes you to shift between stages.

What stage are you in today?

_____

What behaviors or thoughts let you know what stage you are currently in?

_____

What behaviors or thoughts let you know what stage you were in six months ago?

_____

One year ago?

_____

Five years ago?

_____

Describe the factors you believe have stood in the way of your getting into the action phase (for example, fear, lack of time, or stress):

_____

_____

Now that you know how ready you are to change, you can make realistic goals and expectations for yourself. Let's look at the pros of mindful eating, and the cons, the factors that are likely to make you slip back into old habits.

pros and cons of becoming a mindful eater

There are some very good reasons you engage in mindless eating. Logically, you know it isn't healthy or good for your overall self-esteem. However, the mindless overeating or undereating provides you with some benefits that are hard to let go of. You have to be honest with yourself about what you are going to miss about that behavior and the function it plays in your life. In the worksheet below, list at least three pros and cons related to changing your mindless eating habits. An example of a pro might be the following: "Mindless eating gives me a lot of joy: it's fun, it helps me deal with stress, and it allows me to eat good foods." A con might be the following: "It's only fun for a few minutes and it leads to feelings of regret and guilt."

mindfulness pros and cons ─────────────────────

	PROS		CONS

PROS

1.

2.

3.

4.

5.

6.

7.

8.

CONS

1.

2.

3.

4.

5.

6.

7.

8.

These pros and cons will help shed insight into why you hold on to mindless eating habits. Even if you don't like mindless eating, it may be giving you some benefits that are hard to leave behind. That is the ironic part: if you don't enjoy what you are doing, why do you continue? Ask yourself, "What payoff do I get from continuing to mindlessly eat? What payoff will I get from beginning to eat mindfully right now?" Write your answers below:

_____

_____

_____

_____

The Function of Mindless Eating

It's important to get to the root of *why* you mindlessly eat. Most people stop at the surface level: "It tastes so good," or "I just can't stop myself." They obsess about what they eat or don't eat: "I shouldn't eat this cheese-cake," or "I feel fat when I eat candy." But it's critical to know the emotional undercurrent that controls the urge to eat or not eat. Below are common psychological reasons people engage in mindless eating or worry about their weight. Mark the reasons that apply to you.

the function of mindless eating ————————————————

Why I engage in mindless eating:

_____ As a source of pleasure

_____ To zone out

_____ As a reward

_____ To be social

_____ To fill time or relieve boredom

_____ To relieve stress

_____ To get comfort

_____ To cope with negative feelings or thoughts

_____ To numb emotions

_____ To save time

_____ Other: _____

Why I worry so much about my weight:

_____ To improve my self-esteem

_____ To feel in control

_____ To receive attention

_____ To deal with anger

_____ To obtain perfection

_____ As a distraction from other issues in my life

_____ As an excuse ("People don't like me because I am overweight.")

_____ To make me unique ("My identity is being the thin person.")

_____ Out of habit

_____ To look good

_____ To make people like me better

_____ Other: _____

Take a few minutes to reflect on what you learned about what is fueling your mindless eating. Write about it below.

_____

_____

_____

_____

Keep in mind that if you take mindless eating out of your life, you have to replace it with another behavior that fills the same function. So, if you mindlessly eat to fill time or alleviate boredom, you will need to find many activities to keep you busy! If you don't know why you are mindlessly eating, ask yourself, "What function is mindless eating serving in my life right now?"

mindful meals

What is a mindful meal? A mindful meal is generally defined as one in which you pay attention to what you are eating, enjoy it, and feel satisfied, not stuffed or starving. This can take place in many different forms.

For some people, a mindful meal would mean eating at a table rather than at a desk or in a car. For others, a mindful meal is paying attention to the portion size and eating until they are just full. Still others are challenged by letting go of the guilt and actually enjoying the food. A new mom may see a mindful meal as one in which she is able to focus on her own food rather than juggling between feeding a baby and herself. An executive may see a mindful meal as being a hot plate with a vegetable, starch, and main dish that doesn't come from a vending machine and that he doesn't eat at his desk.

Let's spend some time really getting to the heart of what you would consider a mindful meal for your particular lifestyle.

Mindful Meal History

In part, people learn mindful and mindless eating habits from their caregivers. Significant role models in your life don't make or break your eating habits, but they definitely have their place in shaping them. Given this fact, it is important to think about *where* and *when* you ate as a child and its effect on how you think and feel about food today. For example, if you grew up on a farm, perhaps you ate heavy, sit-down meals of primarily meat and potatoes. Or, if there were a lot of children in your home, you may have hoarded food because you had to fight to get your share. If your parents were divorced, you may have been responsible for your own meals and now find yourself drawn to takeout.

mindful meal history worksheet

Describe the setting, types of foods, atmosphere, and length or speed of meals. Did your family snack mindlessly?

_____

_____

1. Describe what meals were like as a child:

    _____

    _____

    Who was present?

    _____

    _____

    Where did you eat?

    _____

    _____

    What was the environment like? Tense or relaxed? Crowded? Messy?

    _____

    _____

    What comments did your family make about food when you ate? Did they talk or were meals usually silent?

    _____

    _____

What kind of relationship did family members have to food? For example, was there a food pusher, someone who urged you to eat a lot?

_____

Did any family members diet? If so, how often?

_____

Did you have family meals, or did you eat alone?

_____

What kind of food did you have access to? Was it nutritious?

_____

What were some of the underlying messages you received about food? For example, did people treat food as a way to deal with stress or as a way to be social?

_____

2.   Describe a typical meal when you were a young adult or teen.

_____

3.   Describe the atmosphere of meals in your current home.

_____

4.   How does your partner's family meal history differ from or resemble your own?

_____

5.   What does your partner expect from your meals together?

_____

_____

mindless overeating and undereating habits

Do you have a nervous habit, a behavior you automatically do when you are worried and stressed? Many of us do. Let's take biting your nails for example. You may not realize how much you bite your nails until one day when your friend asks you, out of the blue, if you are worried. You look at her in surprise. How did she know you were stewing about something? Your friend lets you in on a little secret: she has noticed that you chew on your nails whenever you worry. But you are so focused on your stress that you are not tuned in to it or even aware of what is happening in your body.

In another example, Mary, a twenty-four-year-old schoolteacher, quickly switched the topic whenever her eating habits were brought up in counseling. Until this was pointed out to her, it was an unconscious habit; she didn't divert from this topic intentionally. But changing the subject helped her successfully avoid the anxiety that would come up just talking by about it. Now, when her therapist mentions her eating habits, she smiles and says, "I notice that I want to change the subject, but I'm not going to."

These unconscious nervous habits are very similar to mindful eating. There are times when you have been very aware of how much you dislike mindful eating, but there have been other times when you weren't even conscious of slipping into the same old behavior.

Remember that an important part of changing your mindless eating is to identify the daily habits or routines that stand in the way of your healthy eating. The next two worksheets will help you identify some of the most common habits mindless eaters encounter. The first looks at the typical patterns of mindless overeaters.

tracking your mindless overeating habits

This worksheet outlines various types of mindless overeating habits. Place a check mark next to the kinds of mindless eating you struggle with.

_____ **Multitasking Mindless Eater:** You do another activity while eating (such as talking on the phone, driving, or reading the newspaper).

_____ **Zoned-Out Mindless Eater:** You munch on food while watching TV, not really tasting or enjoying the food. You eat with no real awareness of how much you are eating or how it tastes.

_____ **Emotional Mindless Eater**: You eat when you feel any emotion, whether positive or negative. You eat when you feel joy, excitement, pain, or sadness. People often eat when they are happy to keep the good feelings going. They eat to make bad feelings go away or lessen the intensity of the emotion.

_____ **Restaurant Mindless Eater:** You see eating out as a treat and tend to overdo it when you dine out.

_____ **Time-Clock Mindless Eater:** You eat by the clock, sitting down to eat at 12:00 noon whether you're hungry or not, or having a snack every night at 8:00. You find that you struggle the most with mindless eating at a particular time of day, such as at night.

_____ **Clean-Plate Mindless Eater:** You eat everything on your plate no matter what, or you feel guilty about wasting food.

_____ **Good-Job Mindless Eater:** You use food as a reward or treat.

_____ **Free-Food Mindless Eater:** When there is free food, you always take a bite, whether you are hungry or not and whether you like the food or not.

_____ **Social Eater:** You overeat or mindlessly eat with other people who tend to be mindless eaters. Or, you tend to eat mindlessly when you are at a party.

_____ **Habitual Mindless Eater:** You tend to have routines around your mindless eating, like having a snack while you watch your favorite TV shows every night or picking up a hamburger when you drive to a certain part of town.

_____ **Snack Grazer:** Your meals are pretty good; it's the between-meal snacking or eating a little here and there that adds up.

_____ **Portion Eater:** You feel the urge to eat the entire serving, whether it be a bag, a box, or a bowl. You have trouble stopping before the portion is done.

_____ **Desire-to-Feel-Full Eater:** You worry about not feeling full and sometimes overeat for fear of not being full.

_____ **Multiple-Items Eater:** You like complex tastes. You aren't satisfied by one item of food.

_____ **Second-Helping Eater:** You tend to automatically go for another scoop of whatever you are having.

_____ **Drawn-to-Certain-Foods Eater:** You eat pretty healthy foods for the most part, but you find yourself drawn to overeating one type of food: carbohydrates, sugary foods, or items of a certain color or texture.

_____ **Instant-Gratification Eater:** You see it and you want it. You want the immediate reward of good food.

_____ **The Oh, Well! Eater:** You messed up today so you gave up for the rest of the day.

_____ **Secret Eater:** You tend to eat in private or in secret. You may eat with others and then eat again later when no one is watching.

_____ **Convenience Eater:** You grab what is handy or easy to eat rather than preparing healthier options. This often leads to fast food or snack items.

_____ **One-for-Me, One-for-You Eater:** Parents often describe mindlessly eating their children's leftovers, taking a bite while feeding their kids, or nibbling on a child's or partner's fries.

_____ **Tandem Eater:** You eat the same amount and at the same pace as your dining companions.

_____ **Love-the-Taste Eater**: You enjoy the taste of food so much that you want more of it.

Use this space to summarize what you have learned about your mindless overeating patterns:

_____

_____

_____

_____

_____

_____

tracking your mindless undereating habits —————————————

This worksheet describes various types of mindless undereating habits. Place a check mark next to the kinds of mindless eating you struggle with.

_____ **Habitual Rerun Eater:** You eat the same foods over and over again. Sometimes you stick to foods that are "safe" or don't raise your anxiety level.

_____ **Fast-or-Famine Mindless Eater:** You tend to only eat once a day. Sometimes you say it is because you are too busy but it's really a way to cut out food.

_____ **Mindless Dieting Eater:** You've tried every new diet. You tend to get excited about new methods that claim to help you lose weight quickly.

_____ **Mindless Myths Eater:** You tend to avoid a certain food or foods just because you read somewhere that that food was "bad for you," or you read that a celebrity doesn't eat it, or a friend said that it isn't part of her diet.

_____ **Media Junkie Eater:** You tend to read a lot of fashion magazines, comparing yourself to models in magazines.

_____ **Feeling-Based Eater:** If you feel stressed or your clothes don't feel right, you tend to avoid eating.

_____ **Reward or Punishment Eater:** You tend to eat or not eat if you have been "good" or "bad," which often means that your eating is based on your feeling of being deserving.

_____ **Safe Foods Eater:** You are okay with "safe" or low-calorie foods but tend to restrict certain categories of food, like junk food or dairy.

_____ **Competitive Eater:** You base how much you eat on what other people are or are not eating. If they are thinner than you, it upsets you.

_____ **Dishonest Eater:** You sometimes lie about what you eat.

_____ **All or Nothing Eater:** Either you do it perfectly or not at all.

_____ **Routine Eater:** You have strict routines about how and what you eat.

_____ **Guilt-Based Eater:** You base your food choices on avoiding guilt and have difficulty coping with guilt when you feel that you have mindlessly eaten.

_____ **Secret Eater:** Sometimes, you eat in secret or buy foods that you would not show anyone else.

_____ **Isolated Eater:** You often eat by yourself. Sometimes you turn down invitations to dine out because it is out of your routine and you would have to eat with others.

Use this space to summarize what you have learned about your mindless undereating:

_____

_____

_____

_____

_____

_____

Can I Change These Habits?

Yes! The good news is that these behaviors are just habits. They aren't written in stone. The first step is to just notice any automatic behaviors or daily routines that contribute to the problem. When you catch yourself doing these, just point it out to yourself. Say, "Oh, there I go again doing that habit." So, if you placed a check mark by any habits on the previous worksheets, reassure yourself that it's okay. Begin to pay attention to *when* and *why* the behaviors pop up in your day. Do you fall into this habit because it makes your day easier or faster? Do you fall into the same old song and dance because you are so busy?

Don't worry! Each mindless habit has a mindful antidote. However, it will take some dedicated attention for you to change your routine. The next chapters in this book delve deeper into the seven skills, which provide further detail on how to mindfully approach the problem.

mindful eating contract

Writing a contract is one way to help you alter your mindless eating. Making a commitment on paper helps you to formulate your goals and increase your *awareness*. However, you have to be aware and present with the idea of where you are going in order to go in the right direction. Most contracts are only effective for what you are really willing and ready to do. When I work with my clients, I ask them to draw up their own contracts. A therapist can come up with lots of ideas, but if the person isn't willing, ready, or able to commit to the changes, the contract won't be helpful. Be realistic and start with baby steps. Here are some examples of things people have written into their contracts:

- I agree to have a more mindful attitude.

- I agree to eat more mindfully for at least one meal a day.

- I agree to pay attention to the process of eating.

- I agree to eliminate my diet mentality. Although it feels wrong to let go of it, I will trust that I can stop the fad-diet cycle.

- I agree not to judge my own habits and other people's eating habits.

- I agree to speak mindfully about my food and be aware of when I use words that trigger mindless eating.

- I agree to cut out one mindless routine, like the snack I have every day when I come home from work.

Here's a sample contract:

mindful eating contract ————————————————————————————

I, _____ (name), agree to work on being more mindful of my eating. This does not mean I have to make drastic changes to what I eat. It simply means that I will start paying more attention and being more compassionate and nonjudgmental of myself (avoiding use of words like "I'm bad" or "I'm fat").

I will start working on mindful eating on _____ (date).

I will begin to be more mindful of the following specific behaviors (some examples are written above):

_____

I will reevaluate or renegotiate this contract on _____ (date).

Mindful Eating Goals

The key to setting goals in your contract is to make them *specific, realistic, and obtainable.* For example, instead of saying, "Eat less," think, "Stop eating mindlessly at dinner two nights this week," or think, "Add two mindful meals a week."

Process vs. Outcome Goals

When you are mindful, you focus on process goals rather than outcome goals. An outcome goal is one in which you focus on what you want to happen in the end, such as losing five pounds. This is why frustration occurs: you are more focused on the long-term return rather than what is happening *in the moment.* A process goal includes behaviors that would make the desired outcome happen—go for a walk three times a week, be mindful of my two snacks for today, and so on—anything that you can put on a list and check off today. It helps you to feel good and in charge in the moment.

In the spaces below, write down some process goals that would help you reduce your mindless eating, and keep them in mind when creating your contract.

Short-Term Goals (To Accomplish This Week)

1.

2.

3.

Long-Term Goals (To Accomplish Within the Next Six Months to a Year)

1.

2.

3.

Below are some basic mindful eating goals you might consider:

1. To slow down when I eat. When I eat, just eat. To be fully present, mentally and physically.

2. To be mindful of "picking" at food, or other mindless behaviors.

3. To be aware of *when* I am mindlessly eating.

4. To closely watch my most ingrained mindless habit (eating at night, eating while I drive, or snacking with friends, for example).

5. To clearly identify and catch myself when I start engaging in mindless eating due to emotional triggers.

6. To use a stress ball whenever I get the urge to eat because of emotions.

7. To be able to eat the foods I crave, like chocolate and junk food, in a mindful way.

stepping away from numbers

You might notice that the previous contract and goals worksheets do not give any examples of goals that include clothing sizes or pounds. It's likely that you are tempted to set specific weight-loss goals. This is a common urge for dieters. Before you consider doing this, however, read the following section. It will help you understand the benefits of thinking about your goals in a different, mindful way.

Each of us has a weight range that is natural for our body. However, it's easy to fall into the trap of expecting ourselves to be always at the lowest end of that range. In the exercise below, you will figure out the range that is ideal for you.

being mindful of my natural weight range ───────────────

Lowest weight   **Highest weight**

Part 1

Begin by placing an *X* on the line above to signify where your current weight falls. Are you at your highest or lowest weight, or somewhere in between? You don't need to know exact numbers; rough estimates are okay. Rely on how you feel or fit into your clothing. Then, answer questions 1 through 6 below. Plot the numbers on the line. For example, 1 will be placed on the left end of the range.

1. **Lowest Weight:** This is the least you've weighed in your adult life. (If you are an adult, do not choose your high-school weight.) For example, perhaps your lowest weight was two years ago, when you had a jogging buddy. Write down that weight below, the approximate date, and the circumstances in your life at the time.

   _____

2. **Highest Weight:** This will be the most you've weighed in your adult life. Write that number below, the approximate date, and the circumstances of the time.

   _____

3. **Medical Conditions** (such as pregnancy, reaction to a medication; this includes current and past conditions):

   _____

4. **Ideal or Healthy Weight:** Below, write your ideal weight according to a body mass index (BMI) chart. You can find a BMI chart online at websites such as the Centers for Disease Control and Prevention (www.cdc.gov). Or, if your doctor has specified a goal weight for you, you can use that number.

   _____

5. **Realistic Weight:** A realistic weight is one that your body would likely be able to reach. It's what your weight would be if you were just eating mindfully (not on a diet or starving). Write that number below.

_____

6. **Fantasized Movie-Star Weight**: This is the weight you dream about having, the number that often sabotages you into thinking you are not good enough.

_____

Part 2

Now, in the space below each number on the line, write the date and events happening in your life at that time. Do you notice any trends or reasons your weight shifted? Most people don't go to bed one night and wake up the next day with dramatic shifts in their weight. Often, it happens so slowly it is below their awareness. Looking back helps you to see the circumstances that led to changes in your weight. Write your thoughts below.

_____

_____

_____

_____

_____

_____

Minding Your Relationship to the Scale

It's hard to give people a blanket statement advising what to do with their scale. Some professionals say, "Stay off the scale! Get rid of it." For some mindless eaters, this is excellent advice. The scale determines their mood: a slight change in weight can make or break their day. In fact, dieters are often more mindful of their weight in pounds than their interactions with food. When you are numbers oriented, you often think more about the weight change than the behaviors that are needed to make it happen.

For other people, staying away from the scale is a way of avoiding anxiety. The numbers on the scale trigger so much self-judgment, and they just can't face it. Still others need the scale in order to help them stay accountable and really aware of how much they weigh. These are the people who gain weight and don't even realize it.

minding the scale

What is your relationship with the scale? Do you avoid it? Do you jump on it daily? What habits do you have around weighing yourself?

What kind of emotional response do you have to the scale? Do you feel elated when the numbers drop? Are you devastated and deflated when the numbers go up? Are you numb to the numbers?

What kind of thought patterns do you have in response to what the scale tells you? Do you think about the numbers a lot? Do you obsess about them? Do you avoid the numbers altogether?

How to Mindfully Handle the Scale

1. **Set a realistic schedule.** If you need to have some gauge for your weight loss or gain, and you know that you won't be able to keep away from the scale, set up a time frame and conditions under which you will weigh yourself. For example, you will use the scale every other Monday morning before you get dressed for work. Do *not* weigh yourself more than once a day. If you find yourself on the scale too frequently, that may be the sign of a possible problem.

2. **Lose the scale and use a better measuring tool.** If you have to have some gauge of your relative weight, choose your favorite pair of jeans. Use them as a measure of any changes. The fit of your clothing is actually a better reflection of changes to your shape, and it causes a lot less anxiety than the numbers on the scale. For more specific measurements, use the Body Mass Index chart (again see www.cdc.gov) or a measuring tape around your waist or hips.

3. **Meet with a professional.** If you get too obsessed with numbers or need help keeping yourself on track, enlist the help of your doctor's office or a nurse to chart your weight for you. Take the advice of a professional regarding what is a healthy weight for your body.

4. **Use it as a tool, not a judge.** This is where the mindfulness skills in this book will be of help. For a scale to be even remotely helpful, it can't trigger an emotional tailspin or feelings of elation. Notice and draw your attention to what you feel and think as you step on the scale. Watch and follow your reaction. How does your mood shift as soon as you see how much you weigh? How long does the emotional impact of learning your weight last? A minute? All day?

5. **Focus on a range, not a number.** Never focus on a single number! Aim to be within a five-pound range. Your body is too sensitive to slight changes to stay at a precise weight all the time. Consider your weight to be a rough estimate.

Letting Go of Weight Wishes

Have you consciously or unconscious picked a "magic number," the weight at which you believe everything will be better (you will finally feel on top of the world, you'll love your body, and people will like you)?

Unfortunately, increases and decreases in weight do not fix your emotional baggage. It comes right along with you wherever you go. Anyone who has lost weight can tell you that, despite feeling better about his or her body for a while, it never lasts or patches up all the person's problems. Getting to the magic number is sometimes disappointing. Sometimes it only gives a short reward: you have to lower the number again in hopes of obtaining the benefits you thought you'd receive. Or, after a while, people stop commenting on your weight loss, and you find that you miss the compliments or attention.

What issues do you hope would be "fixed" by your weight loss? It's important to be aware of these issues, because it is very likely that you can deal with each of these issues in a more productive way. For example, if you feel that people will like you better at a lower weight, perhaps you could work on relating to people.

my "magic number" ───────────────────

In the space below, write your magic number. How much do you think you will have to weigh in order to have your problems disappear?

_____

Has your magic number changed? If so, how many times?

_____

If so, why has it changed?

_____

What issues do you hope will be transformed when you get to your magic number?

_____

What is another way you can deal with these issues now?

_____

_____

mindful self-reflection

Now that you've completed the self-assessments, you have a better gauge of your strengths and areas in need of improvement. The questions in these exercises are geared toward stimulating thoughts and reflection regarding your behaviors. Hopefully, it has given you some new insights or at least a direction in which to begin your journey.

Don't forget to acknowledge what you do well, and continue to do more of it! Place the most attention on the skill area you grapple with the most.

You are ready to move on to developing the first skill: raising your awareness.

CHAPTER 4

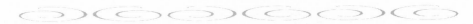

awareness

The moment one gives close attention to anything, even a blade of grass, it becomes a mysterious, awesome, indescribably magnificent world in itself.
—Henry Miller

"What do I want to eat? Every single day, you ask yourself this question, probably many times a day. It may be one of the most important things you think about all day. Sometimes, the answer is very straightforward and simple: "I'd like a blueberry bagel, please." Other times, filling in the blank is unbelievably frustrating.

See if this dialogue sounds familiar.

"Honey, what would you like for dinner tonight?"

"I don't care; what do you want?"

"I don't know. I'm not in the mood for anything particular."

For some people, it is not just hard to put a finger on what they want; it is downright agonizing. They crave a host of menu items all the time. Chips! Ice Cream! Scalloped potatoes! The number of choices and desire for sweets and comfort foods are overwhelming. For some, the urge to eat seems to be attacking from all sides. The question "What do I want to eat?" can haunt a mindless eater all day long.

In this chapter, you will learn to use mindful awareness to (1) identify what you really want to eat, (2) taste food in a new way, and (3) deal with food cravings. Awareness, or tuning in to yourself, teaches you to gently identify what *is* good for you rather than what *feels* good. In other words, awareness is about knowing whether you are really hungry or are having the urge to eat because of an inner temper tantrum.

When your awareness is turned off, cravings and old habits can suddenly take control. When your awareness is on, you can make a conscious decision. (Notice that I said "conscious decision," not "right decision.") Being aware of what you are doing is more than half the battle. When you are just going through the motions, you barely taste what you are eating. You will learn in this chapter to sit down to eat in a new way, and really enjoy food.

how does awareness help?

How exactly can you use awareness to your advantage? How does just focusing your attention on something make any difference whatsoever? It seems overly simple, doesn't it? Let me explain the power of awareness. Let's say this evening you decide to rearrange the clothing in your dresser. You take out all of your socks and put them in a different drawer. What will happen the next time you go to get a sock? It's likely that you will start to reach for the old drawer. That behavior is one you do so often that it's an unconscious habit. Once you open it, you will say, "Oops, that's the wrong drawer."

But, the next time you approach the dresser, you will actively draw your attention to your hand. Before you put your hand anywhere, you will consciously think about where you put the socks and how to direct your hand. In this scenario, you actively place your awareness on your next action in order to get it right. Repeat this for the next week. Eventually, after directing your awareness to the task repeatedly, you can form a new habit. This new habit will soon drop out of your awareness—until you decide to change your sock drawer again.

A similar process happens with mindless eating. Mindless eating becomes a habit, like automatically going to your old sock drawer. Unless you pay attention to your actions, you will do the same thing over and over again in exactly the same way. When you start to eat more mindfully, it takes effort to be aware of the new behaviors, to watch closely when and why you eat. Each time you approach an eating situation, you actively bring your awareness along with you. But, the good news is that once you get mindful eating in place, it becomes an automatic habit that takes less effort.

what is mindful awareness?

Mindful awareness is a little different from the kind of awareness you might traditionally think of. You may think of awareness as the act of simply noticing something. For example, you might notice that there is a chair in the room or that you are stressed out. This is one part of it. But, mindfulness takes awareness one step further.

The attention we are talking about in mindfulness is a special kind that is often referred to as "bare attention." Bare attention is a distant observation of what is happening in the moment, both inside of you emotionally and all around you. You shape your mind to remain open. It is alert and present, contemplating thoughtfully and just watching. However, it watches without judgment. A mindful mind accepts whatever comes into it, regardless of whether it is pleasant or unpleasant. If you find yourself judging, you simply notice that thought. That's it.

You can use this kind of bare attention in mindful eating. With mindful eating, you focus your attention in two ways. First, you tune in to your senses: what you smell, hear, see, touch, and taste. You train your mind to stay present and alert to these sensations. Second, you use awareness as a tool to draw your attention to and be alert to mindless eating patterns. If you observe these patterns without beating yourself up, you will create a productive environment in which you will be willing to work on changing them.

raising your awareness: awareness of *what is*

There are many ways to go about raising your awareness. But you don't have to engage in a formal meditation practice. Instead, turning on your mind so that it is fully alert takes nothing more than the act of being an impartial witness to what is happening.

Your first task is to do nothing. Yes! This is correct. I tell my clients to do nothing different or out of the ordinary at first. In fact, I instruct them not to change one thing in the beginning. Spend a few days just paying close attention to your mindless and mindful eating habits.

I often liken this approach to "people watching," sitting in a public place, like a mall or a restaurant, and just observing the people coming and going. If you've ever engaged in this activity, you've probably noticed yourself starting to wonder more about the people—where they are going, what they are thinking, and what their stories are. In this case, instead of people watching, you are engaging in "self watching." Just observe your behavior and notice the details.

Remember, don't change anything. As thoughts about food or anything else enter into your mind, just notice them. Try not to alter the thoughts. You may notice that you sometimes try to change your thoughts by saying, "Oh I shouldn't think that; I should be more positive." Don't judge the thought ("That is a terrible thought") or analyze it ("I thought that because—"). If you notice yourself trying to analyze or judge, just bring yourself back to witnessing and watching.

For example, let's say you have a craving for chocolate. You say to yourself, "Oh, I notice a craving for chocolate popping up. I saw an ad for chocolate and focused on my mouth, which began to water. I started to think about where I could find some chocolate."

Notice how different this awareness of the craving is from this typical response: "Oh boy, I'm craving chocolate right now. I'm such a screwup! How can I be thinking about chocolate again? Chocolate is a no-no on my diet. If I eat it, I will have

> ## Mindful Eating Tip: *Switch It Up*
>
> According to French collective wisdom, the first two bites of any meal are the best, and everything else after that isn't quite as satisfying. Maybe you've experienced this firsthand. Why is this often the case? It has to do with habituation. Your taste buds recognize the new sensation and then quickly become used to the taste. If you find that you keep eating because you really enjoyed the first taste and are seeking to continue that experience, try switching momentarily to another food. Take a bite of something with a very different flavor, texture, or temperature. If you're eating a hot casserole, take a bite of a cold piece of fruit. If you're eating something creamy, such as mashed potatoes, take a bite of something hard and flavorful, like crunchy carrots. Then, take another bite of the potatoes, or the food you are having trouble walking away from. Do you notice a difference in how it tastes? Varying bites often helps people to slow down their mindless eating.

messed up again." This is an example of how the judgment and evaluation of that craving can sweep you away from your initial reaction—simply being aware of the craving for chocolate.

To obtain this watchful stance, imagine that you are a detective sitting behind a two-way mirror, watching yourself. Like the detective, you will just watch for clues to your underlying motives. You want to discover *why* and *how* you mindlessly eat. You do this by just observing your behavior, thoughts, and feelings.

types of awareness

The way you cut your meat reflects the way you live.
—Confucius

Everyone has a range of awareness in which he or she operates. Sometimes you are probably very focused and almost obsessive about what you put in your mouth. But this hypervigilance often doesn't fit the bill for mindful eating, because it involves judgment and scrutiny. In addition, hypervigilance occurs when you sense danger or are approaching a situation with fear. Think about crossing a busy intersection. You anxiously watch for signs of danger, like a speeding car approaching.

On the other hand, zoning out is quite the opposite. When the mind is on overload and just doesn't want to think at all, zoning out typically follows. Think about eating popcorn while watching a movie: sometimes people will zone out and eat absentmindedly, chomping away at a bowl of popcorn.

Mindful eating offers a middle ground: it doesn't fall into either extreme. It's just the act of noticing what you put in your mouth, without attacking or ignoring.

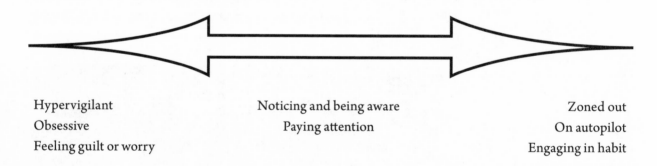

Hypervigilant	Noticing and being aware	Zoned out
Obsessive	Paying attention	On autopilot
Feeling guilt or worry		Engaging in habit

mindful eating exercise: information gathering ——————

You may want to hold off on radically changing your behavior at first. But, if you are anxious to get started, you can invest time in gathering more information. Books and resources can help you to be present and understand your habits in a new way. Basically, the more educated you are about eating problems, the more fully aware you can be regarding the types of thought patterns and habits that are common among mindless eaters. You'll know what to turn your attention to.

For example, a large percentage of people who wrestle with eating issues tend to be perfectionists. They like things to be just so and get very critical of themselves when perfection doesn't happen. Having this information is helpful. You can work on turning your awareness toward perfectionistic thoughts, such as "When I snack, I blow it completely." Also, knowing the connection between perfectionism and eating problems can help you suspend any judgment about your struggle. You can be easier on yourself. You can remind yourself that it's normal (although frustrating) to have perfectionistic thoughts but that it's part of the package rather than a personal failure.

To gain more information about eating issues, read this book and others recommended by friends, a therapist, or your doctor. You may wish to visit www.gurze.net for a comprehensive list of books about eating; this is a great place to find highly recommended books. The creators of the Gurze catalog have done their best to review books and screen out all the wacky and harmful publications out there that claim to be beneficial to people with eating problems. Again, this is just the research phase. Your entire job is to just notice and focus your awareness of how the problem manifests itself. Education helps you to know what to look for.

---

keep a mindful food diary

A great way to raise your awareness of your mindless eating is to keep a food diary. You will learn a lot from this step; don't skip it. Do start this food diary *before* you try to change any of your behaviors, and make sure to continue after you start using the skills. This gives you the opportunity to establish a baseline, rather like a scientist does when beginning an experiment. The scientist begins by simply watching the behavior and conditions as they normally occur, giving him or her a basis for comparison after applying the intervention. Keeping a food diary will let you know if the mindful eating skills are working for you. If keeping a journal is too time consuming at first, try jotting notes on your day planner; keep it in your purse or on your desk. You'll soon get the hang of it.

Four Reasons for Keeping a Mindful-Eating Food Journal

1. **It works!** Research shows that one of the best ways to change your eating habits is to write down what you eat (Hollis et al. 2008). What's interesting is that just simply watching yourself creates improvement. Think about how much harder you work when the boss is in the same room. Just knowing someone is watching (even if it is you) helps you to make changes.

2. **Data collection.** When you have data, it provides concrete evidence of how you are doing. You don't have to rely on your memory, which is often swayed by how you feel at that moment. Notice that this isn't a calorie journal. It's data on your habits and feelings about food.

3. **It's about the process.** It's less about what you write down and more about noticing and keeping mental track of what is going on. Eventually, people stop writing it down and do it all mentally once they get the hang of mindfully observing.

4. **Perhaps you weren't ready last time.** If you are skeptical or keeping a food log hasn't worked in the past, give it one more try. Most weight management programs ask you to track your eating habits. If you've tried a food diary before, it might not have worked because you may have been in an early phase in the stages of change (see chapter 3). However, you may now be ready to dedicate the time and energy required to keep this journal.

I Hate Food Diaries!

Many of my clients feel this way and have shared their struggles with keeping food journals. They find them tedious or anxiety provoking. Does that sound familiar to you? Has this been a part of your struggle? If so, that is okay. If keeping a food journal or writing down your meals makes you anxious, just go ahead and write all about it in your food journal. Use the food journal as a tool to work through this. If you find yourself even fudging the truth in the journal, stop and evaluate why this is so difficult for you. Ask yourself whether you are using the food journal as a place to judge yourself. Have you thought, "I'm so embarrassed; I wouldn't want anyone to look at it!" or "I'm so ashamed of what I wrote down" or "Writing it down makes it worse because I obsess about it more"? If so, it's likely that you are still working on letting go of your inner critic. Remember that writing this down is simply meant to raise your awareness, to put your behaviors under a microscope for observation.

How to Keep an Eating-Mindfully Food Diary

Try keeping a food journal for at least a month, preferably longer. If this sounds too difficult, try just starting with a week and see how it feels. This practice will help you to be more aware of any current patterns. For example, you may find that it is more difficult to eat mindfully on the weekend than the weekday. If writing down what you eat significantly increases your anxiety, just track how eating affects your mind, body, thoughts, and feelings. If you find this helpful, make copies of the blank food diary later in this chapter and continue filling it out for several months. Again, the point is to raise your awareness.

It's a little bit like trying to change your spending habits. If you are trying to cut down on your expenses, you might keep close track of your expenditures by writing it down. Eventually, you will have a good sense of what you spend and will be able to do the majority of the tracking in your head.

There are many ways to structure a food diary. A nutritionist might ask you to focus on the vitamins and minerals you obtain. A diet specialist might ask you to record calories and amounts of food consumed. In this book, we're focusing on the four foundations of mindful eating. When filling out your food diary (introduced later in this chapter), you are asked to pay attention to four aspects of eating—what is on your mind when you eat, how your body feels, and how your thoughts and emotions change when you eat a meal or snack.

It's important to track these four areas, because eating isn't just a physical event. Every time you take a bite, your thoughts, body, mind, and emotions are jolted.

The Four Foundations

The following is a mini guide to the four foundations of mindful eating. Ask yourself the questions posed in each description to help guide what you write in your food diary. If you don't have enough room to write as much as you want, create your own system on your computer or in a notebook.

Mindfulness of the Mind. Think about your level of awareness at this moment. Observe your state of mind, and notice the taste, texture, smell, and sound of food as you eat.

Questions to Consider: How present and aware was I during lunch? Mindlessly munching? Zoned out? Very aware? Obsessed? Attentive to each bite?

Mindfulness of the Body. Listen to your body. Think about whether you pay attention when your body says to stop eating or whether you ignore your body's feedback. Identify how your body tells you it's hungry and full. Tune in to hunger pains, a rumbling stomach, your energy level, movement, body posture, and muscle tension. If you don't respond, your body could stop giving you important information about how hungry or full you are. Specify whether you are experiencing emotional hunger (which may lead to stress eating) or physical hunger.

Questions to Consider: Was I hungry? Did my meal fill me up? How did my body (my stomach, energy level, and so on) feel before and after I ate? Was it what I wanted to eat? How did it taste?

Mindfulness of Feelings. Being mindful of your feelings is noticing feelings that trigger you to start and stop eating. Anxiety, guilt, stress, need for comfort, boredom, and desire for pleasure are just a few emotions that affect eating behavior. It's important to get in close touch with your emotions. Sometimes, identifying and coping with your feelings is just as important as changing the type of foods you eat.

Questions to Consider: How did I feel? Excited? Nervous? Bored? Did I feel satisfied? Was I anxious about the calories?

Mindfulness of Thoughts. Be mindful of your thoughts. Observe "should" and "should not" thoughts, critical thoughts (such as "I'm so fat!"), food rules, and "good" and "bad" food categories. Notice how positive and negative thoughts sway your behavior.

Questions to Consider: What was I thinking about while eating? Were my thoughts compassionate, non-judgmental, or critical?

Awareness of Hunger

We are all born with a natural ability to sense how hungry we are. If you've ever fed a baby, you know what I mean. You can't overfeed a healthy baby. Babies will stubbornly shake their heads no when they don't want to eat any more, and they will cry or give you signs when they want to be fed. If babies didn't have this natural instinct, we wouldn't survive very long in the world.

Somewhere along the way, the natural cues our bodies give us become harder to read. The world teaches us to eat when we aren't hungry. We learn this from TV commercials and from our parents, who may say things like, "You can have this dessert if you finish your entire plate." As an adult, you continue this pattern. You've probably agreed to have lunch with someone, just to be social, when you weren't really hungry. You've probably been offered a second helping at a dinner party even after you told the host, "I'm totally stuffed!" At the same time, diets really encourage people to ignore their hunger level. They tell people to just tune out their hunger, which we all know is such a recipe for disaster!

All hunger isn't created equal. There are different types and levels. Obviously, being a little hungry is very different from feeling starved. Knowing your level of hunger will help you identify how to accurately take care of the situation. If you are a little hungry, a snack rather than a full meal is the perfect antidote.

Use the following hunger scale, which rates hunger between 1 and 10, as a way to raise your awareness, to help you truly listen to your body and hunger. You can begin to retrain your brain to be mindful of what your body *needs* rather than what it *wants*. Aim to start eating when your hunger reaches 6, since it's likely that if you reach 8 you will be at very high risk for mindless eating. As you eat a meal or snack, start slowing down as you begin to approach 5. Some people put a copy of this chart on their refrigerator or pantry door. It serves as a good reminder to check in with themselves before opening the door. If they find that they are at least a 6, they choose to open the pantry or refrigerator door. The more you do this exercise, the more aware you will be of your hunger cues.

For people who diet or undereat, feeling full or satiated can be scary. Diets teach you that feeling full is a sign that you've done something "bad," and hunger can actually feel good because it means that you are doing something "right" by diet standards. Using the mindfulness of hunger scale is a great way to start retraining your mind to trust your body's cues.

On the other end of the scale, what if you feel that you are at 10—absolutely starving—all the time? One reason may be that you have trained your body by feeding it at times when you really didn't

---

Mindful Eating Tip: *Be a Mindful Food Critic*

Many undereaters, dieters, and others who restrict food have trouble enjoying the taste of good food. Why? Sometimes it is because they are so stuck in their head: they are trapped by negative thoughts and fears, and they aren't able to really enjoy the food. Also, pleasure becomes associated with guilt. Dieters often focus more on the worry than on the experience.

If this is the case for you, try taking a mindful bite of a food you used to really love in your pre-diet days. You don't have to eat an entire serving, just a bite. Examine the aspects of this food as if you were a food critic. Try focusing on the taste, texture, temperature, and aroma. Write up a review, or imagine how you would describe this taste to someone else. Next, write another review, this one authored by the dieter inside you. How would a dieter describe the taste? Use your awareness skills to notice whether there is a tug of war between your guilty thoughts and your enjoyment of the food. Identify what thoughts stand in the way of enjoying what you eat. Do you fear that enjoying the food will lead you to feel out of control?

need much food. For example, when you noticed a slight rumble of hunger, perhaps you ate a meal instead of a snack. After doing this repeatedly, your body began to expect a meal each time you were only slightly hungry.

In other cases, there might be another reason, besides a physical one, why food is on your mind all the time. It might be a medical reason. However, when food occupies that much of your thoughts, it is often attached to an emotional issue. Your body and mind are trying to tell you something. You may wish to consult a professional for more help with learning to gauge your physical hunger.

Let's try the hunger mindfulness exercises below and learn about our hunger and fullness.

taking your hunger temperature

With each bite, check in with your stomach. Really get to know the various degrees of your hunger and fullness. Copy this chart and put it on your refrigerator or in another prominent spot.

Mindfulness of Hunger Scale

10 Starving. Ravenous. I feel weak, low energy, and grouchy.

9 Uncomfortably hungry. I am thinking a lot about food and planning what to eat. I feel famished.

8 Very hungry. I want to eat now.

7 Hungry. I could eat a meal.

6 A little bit hungry. I could use a snack.

5 Okay. I feel as if I just ate a snack. I could still eat one or two more bites.

4 Satisfied. I'm not hungry and not too full. Satiated.

3 Comfortably full. I feel as if I just ate a solid meal.

2 Very full. Jam packed. I ate more than I should have. My eyes were bigger than my stomach.

1 Overstuffed. I am uncomfortable. I feel as if I just ate Thanksgiving dinner or another big holiday meal. I feel as if I am in a food coma. My body feels as if it could burst.

Mindfulness of Hunger Worksheet

Now that you're familiar with the hunger scale, you can keep track of the ebbs and flows in your hunger throughout the entire day. It's likely that there are some patterns to the increases and dips in your hunger during the day. After completing this worksheet, take note of the highest and lowest numbers of the day.

Time of day	Level of hunger from 1 to 10	What I did in response to this level of hunger (Ate a meal? Had a snack? Ignored it?)	Was I mindful? If not, how could I be more mindful in this situation?
The moment I woke up			
Before breakfast			
After breakfast			
Midmorning			
Noon			
Before lunch			
After lunch			
Midafternoon			
Early evening			
Before dinner			
After dinner			
Night			
Before bed			
Midnight			
Early morning			
Right before I got out of bed			

Use the Mindful Food Diary to track your daily food intake. Make multiple copies of the blank table, enough for the period for which you intend to keep your food diary. Here's an example of an entry for breakfast:

Meal or snack	Hunger scale	Mind	Body	Feelings	Thoughts
Breakfast *Eggs and toast with butter, juice (8:00 A.M.)*	6	*Very in-the-moment this morning. Paying close attention to taste and process of eating.*	*Very hungry, ready to eat. Body is sluggish.*	*Feeling upset. Scared of fat in eggs.*	*I will be able to think more clearly if I eat instead of skipping breakfast. I often later obsess about what I ate for breakfast.*

Now you're ready to begin your own Mindful Food Diary.

mindful food diary

Date: _____

Meal or snack	Hunger scale	Mind	Body	Feelings	Thoughts
Breakfast					
Snack					
Lunch					
Snack					
Dinner					

am I mentally out to lunch?

> "I'm losing my mind."
> "I was out of my mind at the time."
> "I can't get it out of my mind."
> "My mind is stuck on it."
> "I'm having a mental block."

Have you said any of the above phrases in the last twenty-four hours? To some extent, it's likely that you do track where your mind is at the present moment. But you may only really notice where your mind is when it isn't where it is suppose to be or when you've made a mistake.

Start raising your awareness by tracking where you place your attention when you eat. How present and focused is your mind the moment you pick up your spoon?

mindful eating exercise: mindfulness of mind ──────────

Bring out this scale the next time you eat. Use it to assess your level of awareness. Ask yourself, "Am I really here? Or, is my mind out to lunch?" It's helpful to continue to check in with your state of mind repeatedly throughout the meal. Your focus can rapidly change. Turning on the TV, for example, steals your attention. If you aren't very present at the moment, that's okay. Just ask yourself, "What is clouding my mind? Where am I placing my attention?" You can use this scale in conjunction with the Mindfulness of Hunger Worksheet and Mindful Food Diary, to support your education in being present and in the moment.

Mindfulness of Mind Scale

10 Mindlessly unaware eating. I'm zoned out and multitasking while I eat, unaware of portion sizes (for example, eating directly out of the bag, standing in front of the refrigerator picking at food, gobbling handfuls of popcorn, grazing on food, picking at the breadbasket).

9 Taking big bites, eating very rapidly, finishing everything on my plate despite fullness. Having scattered thoughts. Eating while studying, reading, watching TV, or driving. Being unaware.

8 Very inattentive to each bite. Just eating without checking in with self. Not really tasting the food.

7 Moderately unaware of the process of eating. Eating with little awareness.

6 Occasionally noticing taste, texture, and smell. Fleeting acknowledgment of sensations.

5 Aware of portion size. Momentary acknowledgment of taste and attention to food and body cues.

4 Briefly noticing taste and food sensations. Stopping to place and redirect attention when it wanders.

3 Moderately present in the moment and attentive to eating process.

2 Very alert. Diligently noticing flavors and temperature. Almost all attention is directed to eating.

1 Mindfully aware eating. Completely present in the moment. Aware of every bite. Tasting each grain of salt and smoothness of yogurt. Noticing lifting the fork. Listening to the sound of chewing. Following sensations of food as it travels down my throat. Eating bite by bite.

The Mindfulness of Mind Scale is a great way to become more invested in the process of eating. The next step is to take a mindful bite.

a mindful bite

I watched my daughter take a bite of her ice cream cone. She licked it at a snail's pace and laughed at the sticky dribbles covering her hands. "Mmm," she said as she enjoyed each bite. She pointed out to me each chocolate chip hiding in the vanilla ice cream. I closely watched how she noticed everything. It made me realize that little kids are such naturally mindful eaters. The adult in me wanted to gobble it up. I'm always in a hurry. I hardly notice what I'm eating. Sometimes, I don't even taste it.
—Molly

A mindful bite is the opposite of mindlessly picking at food or grazing, or shoveling in food without really tasting it or being aware of how much you are eating. When you eat mindlessly, you are thinking about the next bite before you've finished the one you have. When you take a mindful bite, you slow down. But don't worry, you don't have to eat at a snail's pace; you just need to eat at a speed that really allows you to taste the food, chew, and swallow slowly enough to notice the spices, texture, and temperature. When you really taste it, you enjoy the food much more and make better decisions regarding what to eat.

Lessons from Eating in the Dark

How important is it to use your senses when you eat? Top chefs believe the senses are the key to a truly satisfying dining experience; they provide a completely different culinary experience. Yet it's hard to teach people to let go of visual cues and just use their tongue to taste a meal. It's so easy to just judge from a single glance whether you will love or hate a dish before you've even tasted it.

There is a new dining trend to remedy this habit: blind dining. Begun with the idea that taking away one of the senses would heighten the others, including taste, blind dining involves eating in the dark. It's caught on in restaurants in various cities around the world. As diners have experienced, eating in a pitch-black environment may increase your sense of taste and therefore pleasure.

mindful eating exercise: eating in the dark ———————————

It is unlikely that you will be eating in the dark anytime soon. However, you may want to try an adapted version of this innovative restaurant idea. If you find that you are having trouble slowing down or just can't stop eating mindlessly, try closing your eyes for a second as you take a bite. For some people, taking away the visual cues helps reduce the temptation to eat everything they see on their plate. Try closing your eyes, and notice how this changes your eating experience.

Hunger is strongly affected by visual cues. As you'll discover, briefly disconnecting from the sight of the food can help break the mindless eating trance for a moment. It can also assist you in taking greater pleasure in what you eat. You may notice a shift in your focus from a desire for more food to the simple enjoyment of the taste on your tongue.

T.A.S.T.E.

When you take a mindful bite, you may find it helpful to think about the concept of *mouthfeel*, a food's physical and chemical interaction in the mouth. When a person is examining the mouthfeel of a food or wine, he or she evaluates the sensation of the food, from the initial perception of its arrival on the palate to the first bite, chewing, and swallowing. With wine tasting, for example, words such as "sweet," "dry," and "tannic," are used to describe mouthfeel, the sensation of the wine in the mouth. Think about how food and wine connoisseurs refine their palates by noticing the subtle distinctions among food tastes. Use descriptive words to label the tastes yourself. Each time you take a bite, give yourself one mindful moment to check in. Use the acronym **T.A.S.T.E.** to help you remember the factors to take into consideration:

Temperature: The temperature affects taste and enjoyment of food. Have you ever eaten a hot cookie right out of the oven? It tastes different than it does when it is completely cooled. Coffee, meat, and soup are often better when they are hot. Use the following words to help you describe the food temperature: "hot," "cold," "scalding," "room temperature," "icy," "boiling," "frigid," "cooled," "chilled," or "burning."

Aroma: It's likely that you naturally take a whiff of a food's aroma before you taste it. This practice dates back to our more primitive days, when early humans would first smell their food to see if it was safe. Even today, you may do the same by smelling a carton of milk to see if it is sour, or sniffing frozen food to find out whether it smells freezer burned.

The majority of what you taste is based on what you smell. People who lose the sense of smell, therefore, have significant difficulty discerning the taste of food. A food's smell can entice you to eat it because of your anticipation of the flavor, or it can drive you away. Deeply inhale before even taking one bite. Notice whether the smell reminds you of anything. Does it spark an emotional reaction? For example, does the smell of cake cause you to think about a birthday?

Speed: How fast do you eat? Do you go at a turtle's pace? Do you slowly chew your food? Are you the last one at the table? Or, are you a speed demon, racing through your meal? Do you feel as if you are gobbling it up at 120 miles an hour?

Texture: A helpful suggestion when tuning in to the taste and texture of food is to find as many words to describe it as possible. Notice that we often lump our entire experience of a food together, calling it simply "good" or "bad." You can work on being more discerning about your tastes. Here are some helpful words: "crispy," "mushy," "crunchy," "watery," "flakey," "crusty," "chewy," "sticky," "hard," "swishy," "slimy," "soft," "creamy," "solid," "silky," "oily," "greasy," "moist," "succulent," "dry," "juicy," and "doughy."

Experience: How does the food taste? Is it sweet, sour, bitter, or salty? Is it spicy? Rich? Delicious? What is your overall reaction to the food? Enjoyment? Displeasure? Surprise? Disgust?

mindful eating exercise: the pretzel ——————————

Choose one piece of food. You might use a raisin, a slice of mandarin orange, or a potato chip. In this exercise, we are using the example of a pretzel.

Begin by looking at the pretzel. Examine the shape, color, and texture. Feel the salt on your fingers as you pick up the pretzel. Take a deep whiff and smell the pretzel, taking note of the aroma of salt. Notice the taste of the salt when you put the pretzel on your tongue. Take a bite, and be aware of the sound of crunching and chewing. As you eat the pretzel, note the rough texture against your tongue. Feel the pressure of your teeth grinding together. Notice how the texture changes as you chew. Now, swallow. Pay attention to the sensations you experience as the pretzel travels down your throat to your stomach. Say the word "pretzel" to yourself in your head.

When you are watchful, you are aware of how your stomach expands and feels fuller. You experience each bite from start to finish by slowing down every aspect of the eating process to be fully aware of each movement, swallow, aroma, and feeling derived from eating. A mindful bite doesn't have to take a lot of time, but it does allow you to connect more closely with your food.

For more practice, choose one piece of food to try in this exercise, such as a raisin, a sandwich cookie, a mandarin orange, or any food that you tend to eat in a mindless way. Write your answers below.

1. When you look at the food, what do you see? What does it look like? Describe the shape and color.

    _____

2. Describe the aroma.

    _____

3. How does the food sound when you bite and chew it?

    _____

4. How does the food feel in your mouth? What is the texture?

    _____

5. Describe the flavor.

    _____

6. Describe the temperature.

    _____

7. What thoughts come to mind when you eat it?

    _____

8. What feelings come up when you eat it?

_____

Remember that it's possible to eat an entire plate of food and not taste one bite. You don't have to do a twenty-minute meditation. Commit to just one mindful bite during a meal.

_____

Mindfully Eating Chocolate

I often teach my clients mindful eating through this classic mindful eating exercise. Some therapists use pretzels, raisins, or oranges in this exercise (I suggested a pretzel in the exercise description above). I give clients a piece of chocolate. Yes, chocolate! I encourage this exercise because I don't believe that the majority of people should cut chocolate out of their lives completely (and most of my clients agree!). Not only would that not be any fun, but it also isn't realistic. Instead of cutting the sugary and fattening foods that we love out of our lives, we should instead learn how to eat them mindfully and in moderation. I am not saying that this will be easy. But because you will encounter chocolate—at parties, on Valentine's Day, and other times—it is worth learning how to eat foods like chocolate mindfully.

When my clients do the mindful eating exercise with one small piece of chocolate, they are often surprised. Here are some common responses:

- "I was surprised by how much pleasure one piece of chocolate gave me. I usually think more is better, but that isn't always the case."

- "I realized that sometimes I don't even finish the first piece of chocolate before I am thinking about and wanting the next one."

- "The chocolate was a lot sweeter and richer than I remembered."

- "The smell really surprised me. It was amazing. I had not slowed down and really focused on the aroma of it."

All of these people described themselves as "chocoholics." After doing this exercise, they were able to gain better control over their consumption of chocolate.

a mindful chocolate meditation

What feelings come to mind when you hear the word "chocolate"? Chocolate can produce a lot of conflicting emotions. We love and crave chocolate, yet many people feel guilty when they eat it. As you do the following exercise, closely notice what emotions arise. Get into a comfortable position. Relax and close your eyes. Use all of your senses.

1. Take one piece of chocolate of your choice.

2. Notice the weight of the chocolate in your hand.

3. Observe the shape and color.

4. As you unwrap it, listen to the crinkle of the foil or wrapper.

5. Touch it and feel the texture between your fingertips as you pick it up. Silently describe the chocolate to yourself: is it dark, smooth, or square? Notice the shape.

6. Roll it around in your hands.

7. Bring the chocolate up to your nose, and inhale deeply. Take a few deep breaths: in and out, in and out. Follow the scent as it travels into your nose and to the back of your nostrils. Inhale and exhale deeply for a few moments. Be aware of what is happening in your mind. Maybe it is anticipation or longing. Let the thoughts come and go.

8. Place the chocolate in your mouth. As you begin to chew, observe the burst of flavor. The richness. The sweetness. Experience the taste. Pay attention to the texture changing and molding to your tongue as the chocolate breaks down in your mouth. Experience the chocolate fully and engulf yourself in the taste sensation. Hold on to the feeling as it begins to fade.

9. Even as you are still eating this piece of chocolate, you might feel a desire, even an overwhelming urge, to quickly reach for another. See if you can relax and stay focused on what you are experiencing in this moment rather than jumping forward and anticipating that next bit of flavor.

10. Roll the chocolate around against the roof of your mouth. Also be aware of any feelings, sensations, or memories of your first bite of chocolate. Maybe it was a chocolate Kiss or bar with crunchy, sweet almonds. Sometimes we feel guilty when we eat chocolate, or we believe a lot of "shoulds" or "shouldn'ts" about eating it. Don't try to push these emotions away.

11. Just be present with the feelings and sensations. Focus all of your attention on the taste and texture. Listen to the sound of your jaw chewing the chocolate and feel the sensation as the chocolate slides down the back of your throat. Imagine the chocolate piece in your stomach. If you are experiencing a desire to have another, finish eating this piece of chocolate, and only then reach for the next to savor. If you don't pay attention fully, you can get lost in the craving.

You've just experienced mindfully eating chocolate from start to finish. Are you surprised that you can obtain such pleasure from a focused concentration on just one piece of chocolate?

Chocolate isn't the only trigger of mindless eating, unfortunately. There are many other foods that you probably struggle with. Changing your relationship with these foods in particular is likely to make a huge improvement in your mindless eating habits.

When clients do this chocolate mindful eating exercise, they often say, "I was able to do it with you, but I can't see doing it by myself. If I were alone, I'd eat half the bag."

They have clearly identified the first problem. If they can't see it in their mind or imagine it, it isn't going to happen. If this sounds like you, before you make any changes to your actual behavior, you have to start with a visualization. If you have trouble eating just one chocolate, try to imagine eating it in a mindful way. Imagine over and over again opening up a bag of chocolates (or a food that you tend to eat mindlessly), taking a handful, closing the bag, walking away, and finishing the pieces you took without going back.

The first time you imagine this, you will visualize what you would likely do without using mindfulness skills. For example, you might have a hard time putting down the bag. You know what you would likely do based on your experiences in the past. Let's now look at what triggers these kinds of experiences.

igniting mindless eating

What gets you started eating mindlessly? Many of my clients tell me that the mere presence of food can trigger mindless eating episodes. Innocently passing a bowl of nacho chips can trigger a desire for them even when that urge wasn't there ten minutes earlier. When food is readily available, it's highly likely you'll eat it—so the presence of food can be a trigger.

Thankfully, not all foods trigger mindless eating. Typically, specific snacks or foods are stronger triggers than others. Chocolate, as we saw in the previous exercise, seems to be a pretty common trigger of mindless eating.

Sometimes these triggers produce a biological response. You may notice your mouth producing saliva and your stomach beginning to secrete juices that are important for digesting food. Other triggers cause unconscious responses. You might find yourself standing in front of the refrigerator or going to the pantry for a snack without even knowing why (maybe you just saw a commercial for pizza on TV). For many people, being too hungry is a common trigger of mindless eating.

Triggers can be tricky to identify, because sometimes they are very subtle: the hint of an aroma, someone mentioning where they went to dinner last night, a twinge of discomfort at work. Other times triggers are extremely obvious. You see a box of cookies and you want them. Your task is to get to know the emotional undercurrents that reliably trigger mindless eating.

Spend some time thinking about the foods you struggle with the most; maybe you are drawn to crackers with slabs of thick cheese, or banana bread. If specifics don't pop into your mind, really pay attention to your reactions to food for a week. When you notice yourself

> **Mindful Eating Tip:** *Mindful Spooning*
>
> In addition to tracking your hunger and fullness, you will also want to monitor how attentive you are to the *process* of eating. How aware are you of what you are doing in the very moment you are eating? Do you notice what you are doing? Do you pay attention to every aspect? Do you notice each handful of peanuts? Do you watch your hand pick up the spoon? Do you notice where you are sitting when you eat?
>
> If you have trouble slowing down while you eat, try putting your eating utensil in your nondominant hand. This will help you become more attentive to the process.

playing the mindless eating tug-of-war over a certain food, where one side of you says, "Stop" and the other says, "No, keep eating," write this food down.

mindless food scale

If You Are a Mindless Overeater, Chaotic Eater, or Mindless Dieter:

Create your own mindless eating scale of foods that are very challenging to eat mindfully. Perhaps potato chips are at 10 on your mindless eating scale while mashed potatoes are at 1.

Most Difficult Foods

Write down your trigger foods and rate them from 10 (most difficult) to 1 (least difficult).

10 _____

9 _____

8 _____

7 _____

6 _____

5 _____

4 _____

3 _____

2 _____

1 _____

Now that you've clearly written these down, start working on your relationship with the foods listed under number 1. Use this food when you are asked to choose a food to work with in other places in this workbook. You will eventually work your way up to number 10. You start with the easier trigger foods because it will be helpful in raising your confidence. You want to teach yourself that you are able to eat trigger foods in a mindful way.

If You Are a Mindless Undereater:

Your challenge, when you are faced with yummy foods, may be different from those faced by mindless overeaters. You struggle more with the idea of eating foods that raise your anxiety or that you perceive as fattening. You may worry about how "bad" the food is. You might obsess about the calories rather than enjoy the taste.

Below, make a list of foods that increase your anxiety. For example, perhaps you love ice cream but avoid it because you worry about the calories and fat in it. At 10 are foods that significantly raise your anxiety. It is hard for you to eat these foods, or you avoid them completely. When you eat them, you feel terrible, so you try to stay away from these items. At 1 are foods that are challenging for you to eat. They raise your anxiety, but not as much as those at the top of the list; you can sometimes eat them without feeling guilty or out of control. For example, perhaps french fries make you very nervous and you never eat them—they are a 10 for you; muffins raise your anxiety too, but you do eat them sometimes—they are a 1 for you).

Most Difficult Foods

Write down your trigger foods and rate them from 10 (most difficult) to 1 (least difficult).

10 _____

9 _____

8 _____

7 _____

6 _____

5 _____

4 _____

3 _____

2 _____

1 _____

Your task is to start learning to enjoy the foods on this list and know that they can be part of your menu in moderation. Start with the foods you rated as 1. Continue to try to do the exercises listed in this book until you become more comfortable with these foods and feel that you can mindfully deal with the anxiety ignited by them. Work your way up to the most anxiety-provoking food. This will take a lot of time. Don't jump ahead of the process. Learn to get comfortable eating foods that push you a little before entering more difficult territory. Doing the exercise in this step-by-step manner will also help build your confidence. As you become successful at mindfully eating some foods, you will show yourself that you can do it!

exercise: being aware of your habits in the moment

Check in with yourself frequently. Don't wait until after you eat. Focus your attention and awareness on what you are doing right now. Just asking yourself, "Am I eating mindfully right now?" will turn your attention inward.

Photocopy this sign and hang it in any environment that tends to prompt mindless eating. Post it on your refrigerator, kitchen cabinets, candy jar—anywhere you need a reminder.

Am I Eating Mindfully in This Moment?

When you check in with yourself, ask yourself whether you are eating mindfully right now. If your answer is yes, congratulations. You are getting the hang of mindful eating. If you are eating mindfully at this moment, it means that you are eating because you are hungry, enjoying your food, eating a portion size that matches your hunger, and tasting each bite.

If your answer is no, don't panic. It's okay! You still have an opportunity to change the situation. Just slow down and investigate the problem.

Make a copy of the sign on the previous page. Cut out the mindful problem solving list below and laminate it. Carry it in your wallet, and use it as a cue card in difficult situations.

Mindful Problem Solving

1. First, identify *why* you are eating. (See chapter 7 for worksheets on triggers.)

2. Try taking mindful bites. (See chapter 5).

3. Take a deep mindful belly breath. (See chapter 6.)

4. See the worksheet on urges (chapter 9).

5. Be compassionate. Remember that you can try again next time. If you do continue to eat mindlessly, remember that you have chosen to do so consciously rather than unconsciously. This is a step in the right direction. (See chapter 8.)

gaining awareness

Now that you have completed this chapter, you may begin to notice that you are developing a budding, new relationship with food. To begin with, you may taste food in a different way. You've started pinpointing some emotional triggers and specific foods that make you feel that you lose the ability to eat in a peaceful manner. All of these exercises aim to help you learn how to clearly focus your mind on the way you choose your food.

You have now taken a significant step forward toward raising your awareness. This is a great accomplishment and an important part of the journey! As you continue your journey, you will learn about the second skill, observation, in the next chapter.

CHAPTER 5

observation

The foot feels the foot when it feels the ground.
—Buddha

In this chapter, you will learn to observe yourself in a mindful way. There are two parts to mindful observation. The first part involves observing what is going on in your body. You learn how to be alert to nutrition, taste, eating the same foods repeatedly, exercise, and sleep—all the physical factors that stimulate your appetite. The second part involves mindfully observing your thoughts. You'll see that you can contemplate what you eat without becoming overwhelmed by the guilty-thoughts monster.

I learned an important lesson in the art of observation in graduate school. When I was a graduate student, I participated in a supervision group in which therapy sessions were videotaped. Afterward, we watched the tape with our peer group. The group's job was to give each new therapist suggestions and to observe body language. Watching the videotapes of ourselves, we saw many behaviors that we had never noticed before. Our eyebrows might scrunch up before asking a difficult question, we might glance at the clock several times, or a foot might bounce nervously. The students' body language clearly showed how nervous they were in session. More important, it showed how easy it is for people to become disconnected from their body movements.

The supervision group took a mindful approach. The group observed the therapist's behavior nonjudgmentally. They gently drew the therapist's attention to things the therapists didn't notice during the sessions, particularly their body language. As the new therapists budded into more experienced counselors, you could see how they incorporated the feedback. They began observing their own body language during therapy rather than after the fact. They stopped nervously bouncing a foot, for example, or if they did it unconsciously, they drew their attention to it and dealt with it in the moment. You can imagine what would have happened if the supervision group had criticized harshly. The therapists-in-training would likely be afraid to go to group each week, and they might even be tempted to avoid it completely or give up.

This is a good parallel to the behaviors mindless eaters engage in when they face their worst critics—themselves. Harsh self-criticism makes mindless eaters want to bury their behaviors and keep them a secret. Or, they avoid thinking about mindless eating altogether. Mindful self-observation is rather like the student group. It is meant to gently place your awareness toward your unconscious habits, the activity in your body that frequently trips you up.

what is mindful observation?

The goal of mindful observation is to see your experience from a distance. This allows you to avoid getting caught up in the chatter in your head. When you get caught up in that chatter, before you know it, you've been whisked away by the thinking, scheming, ruminating, wishing, and agonizing going on in your head.

Food issues are so tricky. They can really do a number on your mind. It's challenging to train yourself to stop listening to and following the demands of your old dieting mind-set. Instead, when you eat mindfully, you work on accurately *describing* what you are doing and thinking, and you hold off on judgment or commentary (such as "I'm a diet reject. I started my diet this morning and have already ruined it, and it's not even noon yet!"). The more you're able to monitor your behavior and thoughts without judgment, the more you prevent thoughts from taking control. You just focus on your body.

Let's move forward with ways for observing the body.

observing the body

A good place to begin working on mindful observation skills is to take a peek at what is going on inside your body. Your body is the best tool you have to manage emotion, hunger, and distress. It gives you all kinds of valuable information. However, observing your body accurately takes practice. Continue to read to find out more about exactly how to do it.

mindful eating exercise: keeping body and soul together ─────────

This is a good time to try a mindfulness exercise for your body. Don't worry, there is no sweat involved! Instead, this exercise requires you to be very still, and it only requires a few minutes. In fact, if you only have a few seconds, that is okay. Some people work their way up to a formal meditation practice. They set aside at least twenty minutes to focus on their entire body. But you can take as much time as you need. It's really up to you.

Begin by just focusing your attention on one part of your body—head, shoulders, or legs. If you want to extend the exercise, it is sometimes helpful to pick a direction. Start with the head and work down, or begin at the fingertips and work inward. Anywhere you would like to start is fine. You may want to close your eyes to block out the distractions in the room, but you don't have to. Your task is to notice any sensations you feel. Is that spot on your body hot? Cold? Tight? Uncomfortable? How does it feel against the chair or your clothes? Does it feel heavy? Numb? Relaxed?

Really try to just be in your body, not your head. Listen to the sound of your breathing. Hear any sounds going on in the room. Sense them without really thinking about them too hard. You may find that it's difficult to stay focused on your body. A to-do list pops into your head and tries to steal away your focus. If this happens, just notice the detour your mind has taken, and return to focusing on that spot in your body.

Another way to focus on your body is to take a hot shower. While showering, if you keep thinking about something that happened at work, just put those thoughts on pause and place your attention on how the hot water feels as it hits your skin. Take in the feel of the soap suds between your toes and the soothing, relaxed feeling of your muscles. You detect the tension melting away as your body temperature rises. As you focus, just feel the sensations happening in your body. Stay with it for a few moments.

Why is this exercise important to the mindless eater? The goal is to help you get less muddled up by your thoughts. When you are aware of your body, you are fully in the moment. This creates an open mind with clearer thinking, and a more focused mind can make better food decisions. For this reason, it's good to get to know your body better under the best and worst conditions.

Check in with your body under several circumstances and at different times of day. Be mindful of your body when you are completely relaxed. Consider how it feels. Also do this exercise when you are feeling pressured or a little stressed. Finally, do the exercise in the midst of a food craving. Place your attention on what your body is feeling under each of these circumstances. When you move your attention from your head to your body, you may notice a shift in your perceived hunger.

If you've got the hang of checking in with your body while you are still, try it when you are in different positions or in motion—while lying down, running, crossing your legs, sitting upright, and so on. Notice your toes pushing against the floor as you walk. Or, place all of your attention for a moment on how the texture of your sweater feels against your skin as you move your arm. These experiences, while simple, will help you become an expert on your body.

mindful eating exercise: all in one breath

There are many verbal expressions about breathing: "A breath of fresh air," "Take a breather," "Breathe easy," "Don't breathe a word," "Breathing new life into it," "He was breathing down my neck," "Catch your breath," "Breathlessly in love." Obviously, the rate and type of breathing you are doing says a lot about your state of mind.

Sometimes the type of breathing you are doing might be the most accurate test of your true feelings at that moment. Periodically throughout the day, do a mini breathing exercise. Stop. Close your eyes for just a second and describe to yourself how you are breathing. Visualize the air going into your lungs and traveling through your body. You don't have to change your breathing; just be aware of its presence. That's it—a pretty easy task. But it can provide you with some valuable information about your emotional state. Here are some common types of breathing to help you describe what you are doing:

- Huffing and puffing

- Can't catch your breath

- Natural, effortless, easy breathing

- Taking shallow breaths (like sleeping)

- Breathless

- Taking deep, slow breaths

- Anxious breathing; short and quick

- Breathing through your mouth

- Breathing through your nose

- Chest breathing—your chest heaves as you breathe

- Abdominal breathing—when you take a belly breath, your stomach moves

- Sighing, as if relieved

- Sighing, as if sad

- Other

You probably notice when other people's breathing styles take a turn; for example, when your partner suddenly starts huffing and puffing. He isn't saying a word, but you are reading his emotions loud and clear. Try to track changes in your own breathing in the same way. Follow the changes in your breathing as your stream of thoughts changes. It's an interesting experiment. How does your breathing change as a negative thought pops into your head? What about a positive thought? A thought about food? About your body?

Mindfulness of the Body

The busier and more stressed out you are, the easier it is for you to lose touch with what's going on inside. You've probably experienced this firsthand. Perhaps you've had a crisis at work and have been so focused on addressing the issue that you completely forgot about lunch. You didn't even realize you were starving until the problem was solved. The busier you are, the more disconnected you are likely to become from your body. But, with mindful observation, you can reconnect. Every time you find yourself unable to hear what is going on inside, use the scale on the next page to perceive what is going on in your body.

mindful eating exercise: mindfulness of the body scale ————

Use this scale several times a day. As you are doing your regular activities, stop and attach a number to your level of awareness of your body. You may wish to choose a specific time or setting each day, such as right before lunch or on your way home from work. The scale will help you gauge how in sync you are with your body. It's helpful to continue to check in with your body frequently. Learn to hear your body.

Mindfulness of the Body Scale

10   I am completely dissociated and disconnected from what is going on inside my body. I don't feel anything. Or, I seem numb or empty. I don't really taste what I eat. I have no idea if I am hungry (or full).

9   I have trouble distinguishing if I am currently hungry or not. I don't trust my body right now to tell me what it needs. I have ignored its signals for so long that I don't know how to appropriately respond to the feeling of physical hunger.

8   I am unsure of what my body is telling me. It feels as if my body and mind send me mixed signals. I can sometimes tell when I need to eat or if I am too tired. I am not too focused on my health or how well my body works.

7   I am out of touch with my body. I only pay attention to certain parts of my body. I often feel as if I sometimes overeat or undereat.

6   I am a little disconnected from my body. For example, I don't always hear my body's cues, like a rumbling stomach, or notice if I feel full.

5   I sometimes hear what my body is saying and respond appropriately to it. If I'm tired, I sleep. If I'm full, I stop. But I'm not doing this consistently, only about 50 percent of the time.

4   I do try to listen to what my body needs and take care of it.

3   I am paying attention to my body's cues. I know when my body should be hungry. I notice as my stomach is filling. I use my body to help me relax. I calm my body through breathing exercises.

2   I am very focused on my body's signals. I check in with my body and assess how it is doing. I know what it needs. I am concerned about how my body works and generally how healthy my body is.

1   I am completely in touch with my body. I hear my stomach rumbling. Changes in my energy level are obvious to me. I notice the posture of my body as it moves. When I pick up a fork, I pay attention to my hand moving. I know my body well enough to be able to gauge just the right portion sizes for me.

Minding the "Just Right" Range

In the tale "Goldilocks and the Three Bears," Goldilocks tries to find porridge, a chair, and a bed that are "just right." Some of the porridge is too hot and some is too cold. Although she undergoes some trials and errors before truly finding a happy medium, Golidlocks is on to something: everyone has to work to find what's just right. So, instead of insisting on *just right,* which implies a judgment, we will focus on getting *just enough.*

You are very aware when you have overeaten. The feeling is often unbearable. When people mindlessly overeat, they sometimes feel sick, bloated, too big for their clothing; it's that "I can barely button my pants" feeling. You are also very aware of when you undereat. You feel as if you could eat a horse, and you are grouchy, lightheaded, and distracted.

The "just right" range is much harder to identify. There are no extremely obvious cues as there are for the other two extremes, starving and stuffed. You have to train your body to tell you when you are satisfied. If you are more familiar with the subtle cues of the "enough" range, you will be better able to know it when you get there.

mindfully full worksheet ———————————————

Write your body's cues in the worksheet below. As you identify additional cues in the coming days or weeks, add them to the worksheet.

Signs Indicating That I Have Undereaten	Signs Indicating That I Have Eaten Just Enough	Signs Indicating That I Have Overeaten

What if I Never Feel Full?

Many of my clients say that they can eat enormous amounts of food yet never feel full. If you don't feel full, it's likely that you've struggled with mindless overeating for a long time. Why don't you ever feel full? It's probably because you have eaten past the point of feeling satiated on several occasions. Overeating can be hard on the body, even dangerous at times. Competitors in hotdog and pie-eating contests can put themselves at risk of rupturing the esophagus or creating a tear in the lining of the stomach, and they do this by training their bodies to ignore the full feeling.

The feeling of being full is hardwired into us, but when you repetitively ignore your body's cues, it stops giving them, or its signals get confused. Think of it like this: Babies cry when they are hungry. This is their way of letting their caregivers know they are hungry and need to eat. Let's say that a parent repeatedly ignores the cries. Eventually, the baby will stop crying when he is hungry, because he knows that his cries won't be responded to. Your body becomes like the baby who has stopped crying. It has ceased sending you messages because you have stopped responding.

Can you change this condition? It's possible. However, it is a matter of retraining yourself to listen very closely to your body's cues. At first, you may not know when you are hungry or full. You may need the help of a nutritionist to create a food plan for you. A professional will show you the amount that would make the typical body begin to feel full. When you eat this amount for an extended period of time, your body starts to send you the correct signals again.

When Do You Stop? Being Mindful of Your *Hara Hachi Bu* Point

Hara hachi bu is a Japanese term meaning "Eat until you're 80 percent full." It originated in the city of Okinawa, where people use this advice as a way to control their eating habits. Interestingly, they have one of the lowest rates of illness from heart disease, cancer, and stroke, and a fairly long life expectancy.

This approach instructs you to stop eating when you feel only slightly full. This is good advice for overeaters who are learning how to fill their stomachs only just enough. Aiming for 80 percent full will likely help you to get a good gauge on this. When you look at your plate, decide how much might make you feel completely full, and then estimate what 80 percent of that amount would look like; perhaps it is two thirds of the food on the plate.

Speed also contributes to mindless overeating. Your stomach takes twenty minutes to digest your food. By that time, you have already left the table. Slow down while eating, and give your body time to register how much you have eaten. If you eat quickly and stop at what you think is 80 percent full, you may actually be 100 percent full and not know it, since your body has not caught up yet with your mind.

The 80 percent approach is also an important skill for undereaters, who may tend to feel too full or bloated when they eat a large meal. Feeling too full is a significant trigger of discomfort, negative feelings, and the urge to purge. If you struggle with undereating,

> ### Mindful Eating Tip: *Find Your Satisfaction Zone*
>
> Let's say you are going to eat some chocolates. It's likely that one isn't enough. You won't feel really satisfied. But eating ten of them, as you may have found out in the past, is way too many. Eating this many has previously led you to feel sick; you can have too much of a good thing! So, the next time you eat too many chocolates (or whatever food you are eating), use this information as a starting point. Try to reduce the number by even just one or two. If ten were too many, are seven "just enough"? Is this a satisfying amount? Continue to practice until you find the comfortable amount.

try eating smaller portions more often to help you to cope with this feeling. Aiming for 80 percent full should avoid triggering the "too full" reaction.

Minus One Bite

Get out of the all-or-nothing mentality with portions. It's hard to leave behind food that is already on your plate, even when you know it might be more than you are hungry for. If you frequently find yourself mindlessly eating portions that are too big, start by just leaving one bite behind on your plate! Then, once you have really got the hang of it, try two bites. But, don't do this until you get comfortable with leaving behind one bite. It's easier to scale back in baby steps to a portion that meets your hunger than it is to begin by cutting portions in half. Pay attention to your thoughts and your body's response to this approach.

physical hunger vs. emotional hunger worksheet

Hunger versus Hunger—it sounds like a legal case, doesn't it? What I'm talking about here is actually physical versus emotional hunger. A big part of mindful eating is knowledge of the difference between hunger that arises from your body and hunger arising from your heart. Bodily hunger comes from your need for nourishment to keep your body going. At bare minimum, you need calories to make your heart beat, eyes blink, and limbs move. Emotional hunger arises from a need to feel better (or feel something). Eating feels good, so it can take away pain or lengthen a pleasurable feeling. Many mindless eaters describe feeling empty. It's this empty emotional feeling that mimics physical hunger—but they only realize it is not hunger when they turn to food and it never seems to fill up that hole.

List the symptoms of *physical hunger* (for example, you have a rumbling stomach, you realize it's been several hours since your last meal, and so on):

_____

_____

_____

List the symptoms of *emotional hunger* (for example, you just ate recently and you find yourself scrounging in the refrigerator):

_____

_____

_____

The next time you eat, remember to mindfully ask yourself, "Am I physically hungry or emotionally hungry?" If you are physically hungry, that's fine. Have a snack. If not, identify the feeling and deal with it accordingly. If you are tired, take a nap. If you are lonely, call a friend. Do not allow yourself to get too hungry. Being overly hungry or starving is the number one reason people mindlessly overeat. (See the "Mindfulness of Hunger Scale" in chapter 4.)

Foods That Help You Feel Physically Full

Consuming fiber, whole grains, protein-rich foods, and water can help your internal sense of feeling full before your stomach is overfilled. Salads with lots of vegetables, soup, and fruit all have a high water content and therefore can help you feel full sooner.

A great book for people who struggle with feeling full is *The Volumetrics Eating Plan: Techniques and Recipes for Feeling Full on Fewer Calories* by Barbara Rolls (2005). A professor at Pennsylvania State University, Rolls is well known for her research on the way people eat and how much they consume. In general, her research leads to many important findings: we tend to eat according to volume, or how full we feel. We judge how much to eat based on how full we feel rather than how many calories we think we've consumed.

This makes a good case for being a deceptive chef. The more you can bulk up the volume, or amount of your meal, with low-calorie items, the better. For example, you might throw a bag of vegetables in with a bowl of macaroni and cheese. Think about how this step increases the volume of food to help you feel full without sacrificing the overarching taste or adding calories. This approach is quite different from, and possibly much easier to achieve than, the "simply eat less" idea.

Another example might be a pizza with vegetables and less cheese rather than a pizza made with several meats. Four pieces of veggie pizza, a much bigger volume, equals the approximate calories in one to one and a half pieces of meat pizza. If you have trouble eating just enough but not too much, trying out the recipes in Rolls's book may be a good experiment for you. Again, remember that trying these recipes is an effort to cut or obsess about calories. No way! The point is to help your body send clearer cues about fullness that you can recognize easily.

> **Mindful Eating Tip:** *Make Your Eyes Smarter Than Your Stomach*
>
> Don't let your eyes deceive you. You might be eating more than you think.

Managing Portion Sizes

Brian Wansink, the author of *Mindless Eating: Why We Eat More Than We Think* (2006) and a professor at Cornell University, has done a number of studies on portion control that have repeatedly found that people are pretty poor judges of how much they eat. They often unintentionally and unknowingly consume much more than they think. In his book, he discusses a number of intriguing studies that proved this fact.

For example, in one of these studies, Brian Wansink and Matthew M. Cheney (2005) found that bowl sizes can be pretty sneaky. Even the size of the serving bowl, something we really don't think much about, can affect how much people consume. In their study, they invited people to a Super Bowl party. Some of the guests were directed to a buffet table that had snacks set out in large bowls. Other people were directed to a table that had identical snacks but in smaller bowls, about half the size. The people in this study served themselves.

According to their findings, the serving dish made a difference in how much the participants consumed. People who served themselves from a large bowl consumed 56 percent more than did those who served themselves from small bowls. Apparently, what is next to the food and how it is served affects how we *see* the portion size and how much we think we are eating. It is like judging whether a five-foot-seven-inch-tall person is actually tall by comparing him or her to a professional basketball player or a child.

Clearly, it's a good idea to think about how food is prepared and served. So grab a larger bowl for healthy foods and a smaller one for desserts. See www.mindlesseating.org for additional clever studies on the way portions urge you to eat mindlessly.

What else do the findings of these studies suggest to mindless eaters? That they have to carefully use their eyes. Studies like these suggest that is very hard not be tricked, even when you are mindful of your environment. You have to be continually watchful for things that may trip you up—even the way you serve yourself food. Everything, including the type and size of dishes you use, influences how you eat.

mindful eating exercise: mindful portions ————————————

Do a self-experiment. Get out two bowls, a large one and a small one, and a box of breakfast cereal. Put one of the bowls out of sight for a moment, and pour into the other one the amount of cereal you think you would be likely to eat on an ordinary morning. Put this bowl out of sight, get the other bowl, and pour cereal into it, with the same intention. Place as much as you think you would eat into it. Then get both bowls and measure the amount in each. Is it exactly the same? It's likely that there is probably a bit of a difference.

Mindfulness of Yield Signs

Imagine you are driving in your car. You approach an intersection with a yield sign. What do you do? As you approach the sign, you don't stop. Instead, you just slow down and cautiously approach the intersection. You look back and forth carefully, watching for any unforeseen danger. Eating mindfully is similar to seeing a yield sign. You don't stop eating; you cautiously look around for signs to continue or stop eating.

Many of my clients describe being unable to stop once they've opened a bag of pretzels or cookies. They just keep going until they reach the bottom. Big bags, particularly those you get from discount or warehouse club retailers, are dangerous because of their size. They don't help people to yield or slow down.

You can make your own yield signs. When you snack or eat a meal, visualize a yield sign popping up. Imagine the yellow, triangular sign hanging right above your plate. Slow down. Look around for signs of danger that you are approaching a mindless eating zone. Visualization works well for many people, but if imagining the sign doesn't work for you, you can build in more tangible yield signs, as outlined below:

Dish out portion sizes in little baggies. Take a large bag of pretzels and divide the contents of the entire bag into sandwich-bag-size portions. When you get to the bottom of one of these small bags, you are forced to ask yourself if you are still hungry. If you determine that you are still hungry, feel free to open another bag. Dividing up the big bag reminds you more frequently to check in with your hunger and ask yourself if you really want more.

Putting snacks into a sandwich bag is also a very helpful strategy for undereaters who fear that if they start eating they will lose control. Having a variety of snacks packaged in reasonable portion sizes and ready to go can remind you that it is okay to eat a snack. It can also ensure that you are eating a correct portion size, which allows many undereaters to feel more at ease.

During a meal, imagine a yield sign each time you take a drink. Make sure you take many sips! Imagine that your drink is a yield sign, urging you to slow down, take a closer look at your plate, and see if you are actually hungry enough to continue eating.

my yield sign is . . .

Describe your own strategy here:

_____

_____

_____

_____

_____

_____

Mindfulness of Nutrition

Good nutrition is the key to good health, preventing disease, and promoting healthy growth. In order to be mindful of your body, you need to raise your awareness of what you put in it and how it affects your body's functioning.

nutrition worksheet

Ask yourself the following questions, and write the answers below:

1. Do I get a variety of foods (fruits, vegetables, proteins, fats, and so on)?

   _____

2. What foods do I seem to miss out on (green vegetables, for example)?

   _____

3. Is there a type of food I eat out of balance, or more or less of (such as meats and carbohydrates)?

   _____

4. Is there a food group I completely avoid?

   _____

5. Why don't I eat a healthy balance of foods? Check all that apply below.

____ I am fearful of certain foods.

____ My diet says certain foods are a no-no.

____ There are certain foods I don't like.

____ Particular foods don't taste as good as the foods I do like.

____ Some food is not convenient or available.

____ I avoid foods that I don't know how to cook.

____ The foods are expensive to buy.

____ I don't think I need certain foods.

____ I've never thought much about nutrition.

____ I'm a picky eater.

____ I'm allergic to certain foods.

____ I've not been exposed to certain foods.

____ Other _____

6. How does the lack of balance in my nutrition make me feel (for example, it doesn't make much difference, or I feel exhausted when my blood sugar dips in the afternoon)?

_____

7. If I were more mindful of nutrition, my number one goal would be:

_____

An imbalance of nutrition can dramatically affect how well your body functions. For example, you might blame your low energy on everyday stress or lack of sleep. Occasional low energy is normal, but if it is an everyday occurrence, nutrient deficiencies may be the culprit. For example, consider the symptoms of iron deficiency:

- Feeling tired and weak

- Decreased work and school performance

- Slow cognitive and social development

- Difficulty maintaining body temperature

- Decreased immune function, which increases susceptibility to infection and illness

Ironically, all of these symptoms could stand in the way of your developing healthy eating habits; mindful eating is difficult when you feel weak or your temperature isn't regulated.

mindful eating exercise: holding it ————————————————

Sometimes, but not always, you get a sense of how healthy a food is by just holding it. Have you ever held a sticky cinnamon bun or felt the wrapper of a greasy burger? Just tuning in to the way food looks and feels in our hands might affect how we eat it.

Take a moment to touch whatever it is you are eating. What impression does it leave you with? If it is a grape or candy bar, roll it around in your hand. Feel the texture. Take note of the consistency. Describe the texture and sensation to yourself: rough, smooth, meaty, or grainy? What does the feel of it tell you about this food? What does it suggest about the quality? For example, many people find that they are turned off by greasy foods when they really pay attention to how these foods feel in their hands.

A Mindful Eating Experience

It can be difficult to be mindful in familiar surroundings, but you are often forced to be more aware when you enter a culture other than your own. When your surroundings are foreign to you, you realize you can't depend on autopilot anymore. For example, if you've ever driven in a country where everyone drives on the "wrong" (or other) side of the road, you know what I mean. Instead of driving on autopilot, you become very aware of what you are doing. You notice how you shift gears, and you put great effort into changing lanes, a behavior that requires little thought at home.

Similarly, one of the most mindful eating experiences you can have is to eat foods from other cultures. On my trip to promote the release of *Eating Mindfully* in Japan, I had the good fortune of visiting a monastery, where they served vegetarian cuisine called *shōjin ryōri* (*shōjin* means "devotion," and *ryōri* means "cuisine"). The meal was served on a table about eight inches off the floor, and I sat cross-legged on thin cushions to eat it. The food was elaborately presented on numerous little dishes the size of a saucer and served on a tray. Each plate contained approximately one bite of food. The menu consisted of vegetables, two kinds of tofu, miso soup, pickles, a savory custard, and

> ### Mindful Eating Tip: *How Nutritious Is My Food?*
>
> Be mindful of food labels! We are often unaware of what we are really eating. Top nutritionists advise that we pay attention to the first five ingredients listed on every food label. (Notice that this is different from obsessing about the calories listed on the label.) In an effort to be mindful of what she was consuming, one of my clients went by the rule of thumb that she didn't eat the food if she couldn't pronounce what was listed in the ingredients.
>
> Sugar, enriched flour, and partially hydrogenated oils (like trans fat and palm oil) are three ingredients that have low (and sometimes detrimental) nutrient value. If any of these items is one of the first five ingredients listed, notice how these foods affect your mind and body. Ask yourself, "Is this a snack I have trouble eating in a mindful way?" Many of my clients talk about the fact that eating snacks and meals with these three ingredients can significantly cloud their awareness. These ingredients, more than others, seem to cultivate craving and mindless eating. Now ask yourself, "How does my body feel, and how is my ability to be mindful influenced, when I eat healthier foods, like fruits, vegetables, and breads with 100 percent whole-grain flour?"

rice. Dessert was two poached plums. With each bite, I noticed that I was very mindful, partly because each food was not identified, and it was not obvious what the menu item was by sight. As a result, I had to rely on the taste and texture in order to identify it.

mindful eating exercise: expanding your eating horizons ——————

Try the following exercise to create a mindful eating experience today.

1. Choose an international food that is unfamiliar to you: Indian, Chinese, Thai, Latin, Japanese, Ethiopian, or other cuisine. Go to a restaurant that serves the food you have chosen, or choose a recipe from that type of cuisine (visit your grocery store's ethnic foods section).

2. Order (or prepare) something that is unfamiliar to you in taste and texture.

3. Take mindful bites. Describe the flavor to yourself. Consider how it tastes compared with other meals you are familiar with.

4. Is it easy or difficult to eat this foreign food in a mindful way? Describe your experience:

Mindless Repetition: Food Reruns

Have you ever eaten pizza three days in a row? It's not uncommon for people to get into a serious food rut. The benefit of this restricted menu is that it makes eating and cooking mindless and simple, and it allows you to avoid the many choices that can make you feel overwhelmed. The downside is that it's easy to act on autopilot and get stuck in mindless repetitive eating habits.

List the foods that show up on your menu every single day. For example, perhaps you eat cereal every day for breakfast (maybe even the same kind), and you always have a sandwich for lunch. After you list typical menu items, note whether you eat these foods in a mindful or mindless way.

List the foods you tend to eat repetitively:

How can you add more variety to your daily menu? Here are three tips:

1. **Mindful Shopping:** The next time you go grocery shopping, make a goal to buy just one item that you've never bought before. Pick an exotic fruit or snack. You might need to give yourself extra time at the grocery store to look around for something new.

2. **Mindful Colors:** Choose foods of many different colors. For example, some people overload on white items (such as bread, cereal, or potatoes). Vegetables and fruits add a rainbow of colors and nutrients.

3. **A Mindful Food Plan:** Make a weekly food plan. Hang the plan on your refrigerator. When you have a planned strategy for what you are going to eat that week, you are less likely to turn mindlessly to the old standbys.

Mindfulness of Taste

Filling up on processed and sugary foods can tamper with your taste buds. Our bodies are trained to recognize foods that are grown in nature. The body isn't wired to recognize artificial and chemically engineered products.

When mindless eaters begin to eat healthier, many people complain that the foods seem bland, but that is simply because their taste buds have gotten used to the overbearing taste of processed, sugary, and salty foods. As a result, when we come into contact with more natural foods, we don't experience the same instant gratification. A higher level of awareness and self-observation is needed.

When you switch from whole milk to skim milk, you may do so slowly. You may go from 2 percent to 1 percent to skim. The change is slow and it helps you adapt to the new taste. However, if you take a swig of whole milk after many months of drinking skim, it tastes like heavy, rich cream. Many people can't go back because it is now too rich. The same happens with lemonade. Say you begin to put less and less sugar into each pitcher you make. Later, if you make it with the full recommended amount of sugar, it tastes way too sweet.

When people start to pay more attention to the taste of food and begin eating healthier, they become aware of feeling sickened by foods that are too sweet, processed, or greasy. One of my clients switched from her favorite cereal, which was sweetened, to a similar cereal with less sugar. When she went on vacation, her healthy cereal was not an option, so she ate her former favorite cereal and was shocked to learn that the sugary taste was now very pronounced—something that had escaped her awareness in the past.

The same thing happens in the opposite direction for mindless undereaters. They become so used to bland, tasteless diet food (stripped of any real

> ### Mindful Eating Tip: *Mindfully Adapt*
>
> If you want to make healthier food choices but you are someone who clings to the taste of food, try doing little experiments. Work your way gradually toward healthier, less-processed foods in a step-by-step manner. For example, if you find that you are addicted to sugary cereals, check out how much sugar is in your current cereal. Find one with a gram or two less sugar. After you get used to that one, try switching to one with another gram less. Often people make too sudden of a jump, and the leap is too big for their taste buds to handle. But, when you do it slowly, your body and tastes adapt and you hardly notice it.

substance) like nonfat muffins and low-calorie butter that they forget what real food tastes like. When they take a bite of regular food, they realize that they can't live on tasteless substitutes and artificial sweeteners forever. One of my clients, for example, ate a reheated frozen chicken entrée every day for lunch. She described it as a freezer-burned, tasteless, rubbery substance that resembled meat drenched in a gooey, flour-like sauce. After having a bite of real baked chicken, she became aware of the terrible taste of her regular lunch and was never able to eat it again.

Consider these questions:

What tastes and flavors are you drawn to? Are you a person who likes salty, sweet, or fried foods? If you don't know, think about your favorite snack. Describe your thoughts below:

_____

_____

_____

_____

Describe the way in which mindless eating or dieting has changed your taste or craving for certain foods (for example, you don't like cheese anymore, or you crave sweets):

_____

_____

_____

_____

_____

Mindful Sleep

What does sleep have to do with managing your weight? There is actually a significant relationship between the quantity of sleep you get and the tendency to mindlessly overeat (Prinz 2004; Taheri 2006). So, one of the easiest things you can do to help manage your weight may be to get a good night's sleep. Sounds pretty good doesn't it? Lack of sleep interferes with the delicate balance of hormones that regulates your metabolism and weight.

In addition to disturbing your digestion, lack of sleep clouds your awareness. When you are sleepy, it's hard to focus on anything besides getting in bed. Also, many people mistakenly turn to food to get a burst of energy rather than take a nap or go to bed early.

What is considered to be a "good night's sleep?" That depends on things like your age and health. However, in a recent study, the hormones of participants who slept less than eight hours a night were off balance. They also had a higher level of body fat. Study participants who slept the smallest number of hours per night weighed the most (Prinz 2004).

mindful sleep patterns

Ask yourself the following questions:

- Do I use any substances that interfere with sleep, such as caffeine, cigarettes, and alcoholic beverages, right before bed?

- Do I have a positive sleep environment (meaning that the bedroom is used for sleep only, has a comfortable temperature, no TV, and soft sheets)?

- Do I have a positive bedtime routine?

- Do I have any medical conditions that affect my sleep, such as sleep apnea?

- Do I fall asleep easily? If no, why not?

- How many hours of sleep do I get?

- Do I usually get an adequate amount of rest (approximately eight hours)?

- What factors stand in the way of restful sleep (for example, emotions such as worry, or environmental factors like a late-night work schedule)?

It is my hope that these questions stimulate some thoughts about your sleep patterns. If you have a chronic tendency to eat mindlessly at night, you might have an eating disorder called night eating syndrome. To find more information about this syndrome, please see the online resources section at the end of this book and read *Overcoming Night Eating* by Kelly C. Allison, Ph.D., Albert J. Stunkard, MD, and Sara L. Their.

mind over mood: the mind-body connection

Knowing your body is incredibly important. It's been the primary focus in this chapter. But you can't forget about everything from the shoulders up. What you think affects how you behave. Therefore, how you think about food affects how you eat it. Negative thoughts can be almost as damaging as a tray of doughnuts. You can often see the evidence of this in people who are chronically stressed. The impact of stress alone starts to break down their bodies. They get sick. You might even see a few gray hairs pop out. People who are emotionally healthy are aware of their thoughts, feelings, and behavior. They pay attention to the strong mind-body connection and do what they can to heal both simultaneously.

The following section is intended to help you observe your thoughts. It contains exercises that will help you closely watch your thoughts, which in turn promotes healing in the body. You'll notice the benefits by closely observing your thoughts over time.

Mindfully Observing Thoughts

Seeing things from above or from a distance is one way to think about the skill of observation. Most of the time, our heads are only a few feet off the ground. Our problems seem like giants when we are stuck in the middle of them. Think for a moment about how things look from the window of an airplane. As you ascend into the sky, you watch the houses shrink into doll-house-size objects. The world looks different when you aren't enmeshed in the middle of it. So, the next time you feel overwhelmed, try distancing yourself from the problem for a moment. Take a look at the situation from a different perspective. Instead of seeing it from your own eyes, imagine what it would look like if you were looking down on the issue from far away. This will allow you to see the problems for what they are, and you will be better able to solve them effectively. A good way to practice seeing things from a distance is to watch the cues that control the way you eat.

Mindless Eating Cues

How do I know when I am *done* eating? Mindless eaters often follow certain cues that tell them loud and clear to stop eating. Unfortunately, these stop signs often come too late. For example, when the check arrives at a restaurant, this might signal that the meal is over. However, it is likely that you were full before this point. People learning to eat mindfully change the scripts they follow. Below is an assortment of external and internal cues that indicate the end of a meal:

External Cues:	Internal Cues:
Everyone leaves the table.	Body feels full or satisfied.
The plate is empty.	Stomach feels extended.
The check comes.	Clothing feels tight.
Lunch hour is over.	The conscious thought pops up, saying "I'm done."
Someone starts clearing the table.	The meal seems to have gone on for a long time.
"I have completed my meal plan."	Feeling of guilt appears.
"I have eaten as much as I allow for the meal or snack.	You feel that you have eaten a similar amount other times.

As you can see, you have unconscious cues that tell you to start and stop eating. You might follow these as scripts. For example, you may not consciously say to yourself, "I feel guilty for eating this cheeseburger; I have to stop eating." You may just notice yourself feeling guilty and automatically putting down the burger. This is an example of a cue; guilt means stop eating.

cues that indicate "start eating" and "stop eating" ———————

Take a few moments to reflect on what cues you may be following. If you aren't sure, try working backward. Once you start or stop eating, ask yourself what prompted you to do so. Then, write about it.

Thoughts or events that prompt me to *start* eating (for example, "I sit down at the table" or "I open the fridge"):

_____

_____

Feelings that prompt me to *start* eating (for example, "I feel bored, stressed, or angry"—scripts that lead to automatically acting on the impulse to eat):

_____

_____

Thoughts or events that prompt me to *stop* eating (for example, "I can't eat that—it's so fattening! If I eat that, I blow my entire diet"):

_____

_____

Feelings that prompt me to *stop* eating ("I feel anxious," "I feel heavy," or "I feel motivated to make a change"):

_____

_____

_____

There are lots of times when we act in scripted ways. For example, when you come to a stoplight, you automatically follow its cues. You become more aware of this scripted behavior when the stoplight does something you weren't expecting, like flashing a green arrow. As is the case in this example, scripts sometimes help us. But sometimes they keep us trapped in a cycle of repetitive behavior that isn't working.

Taking a Step Back: Seeing Your Thoughts from a Distance

Mindfulness teachers have come up with several imagery exercises to describe the process of observing thoughts (Kabat-Zinn 1990; Linehan 1993). As I described previously in the example of seeing the world from the perspective of an airplane, the idea here is to see your thoughts from a distance. It's easy to get so caught up in them up close that you forget to take a step back. In fact, just because you have the thought doesn't mean that it is a *true* thought or one that you have to act on. For example, just having the thought that you are fat doesn't mean it is true, and just thinking "I must diet" doesn't mean you have to do it.

Your thoughts can either help or hurt the situation. Often, mindless eaters don't know what to do with destructive, sabotaging thoughts; they obsess or can't seem to let them go, as hard as they try. If you are experiencing these kinds of thoughts, instead of trying to get rid of them, try accepting them (because you can't magically wave a wand and make them go away). Then, just notice them without responding or reacting to them. (For example, you can have a thought about restricting food or bingeing without acting on it.) Try the exercise below to identify your problematic thoughts and automatic responses.

mindful eating exercise: minding sabotaging thoughts

1. Notice the thought. Describe it.

    _____

    _____

2. Ask yourself, if I automatically *reacted* to this thought, how would it affect my actions?

    _____

    _____

3. If I were thoughtfully *responding* to this thought, how would it affect my actions?

    _____

    _____

letting thoughts go

Imagine sitting next to a stream and watching leaves float by. On each leaf is sitting a mindless-eating thought, a judgment or worry about weight or calories. Watch each leaf drift slowly downstream. Observe one thought at a time as it drifts by, and then let each leaf sail out of sight. Return to gazing at the river, waiting for the next leaf to float by with a new thought. Think whatever thoughts come to mind and allow them to flow freely, one on each leaf. One by one down the stream. Allow yourself to take the perspective of the stream. Hold each of the leaves and notice the thought that each leaf carries as it sails by. Just let them flow.

In the spaces below, write what you have discovered about these thoughts.

What thoughts are you having trouble letting go of?

_____

_____

What do you gain from obsessing?

_____

_____

What do you fear will happen if you let go of the thoughts?

_____

_____

_____

Some therapists instruct you to observe your thoughts as if you are watching clouds drift by you. Others use the imagery of a conveyor belt carrying boxes down the line. Each box contains a thought and you simply watch the boxes travel past you without taking any off the conveyor belt (Linehan 1993). Each of these metaphors conveys the same message: Just watch. Observe. Notice what you are thinking.

Outlined below is another metaphor that may help you to conceptualize your observation of your thought patterns and automatic beliefs.

mindful eating exercise: a mindful train of thought

The Shinkansen are Japan's world-famous bullet trains, which go as fast as 188 miles per hour. Imagine that you are just about to cross a railroad track. The guard rails have just gone down. The red lights are blinking, letting you know that the high-speed bullet train is coming. Now, think of the train as being like your train of thoughts. It is sometimes speeding and other times going very slow, but it keeps chugging along. Your temptation is to stop the train of thoughts, or you may even get on the train and become distracted by where it is going (analyzing, believing, reworking, or trying to eliminate the thoughts on the train). It's hard to just let the thoughts go by; it's challenging not to take each thought you have and react to it.

However, just watch the thoughts travel by you as if you were observing them speed by behind the railroad crossing gates. Notice your "train" of thought. Describe your thoughts as they go by. Some of the cars might contain passengers, or people you are thinking about. Other cars might be labeled as "old baggage," with things from your past that you regret. Describe your experience of letting the train of thoughts go by.

_____

_____

_____

_____

_____

_____

The train exercise is about letting your thoughts go. The goal of the next exercise is to label and describe your thoughts. When you label thoughts, it again helps you to see them from a distance. It may be the *type* of thought you are having that is getting you stuck and unable to move forward toward mindful eating.

mindful eating exercise: the sticky notes ————————————

You will have more awareness of your thoughts when you begin to understand the *way* you think. Imagine that you have a pad of sticky notes in front of you. As a thought pops up in your mind, imagine writing the name of the type of thought (see below for a list of thought types) and sticking it on that thought. Some of the thoughts will have more than one sticky note. For example, perhaps the following thought pops into your mind: "I'm a loser because I just can't get my mindless eating under control." You would put several sticky notes on that statement, since it is a judgmental, negative, untrue, extreme thought.

Here are a few thought categories:

- A negative thought

- A positive thought

- An automatic thought, or one that comes to mind unconsciously, without effort

- A feeling thought

- A judgmental thought

- A random thought

- A harsh thought

- A compassionate thought

- A false thought

- An extreme, or black-and-white, thought

————————————————————————————————————

There is a Zen story that nicely sums up this chapter on observing the body and thoughts:

A Zen student was bragging about his teacher to another student. He claimed that his teacher was capable of all sorts of magical acts, like writing in the air with a brush; he said that the characters would appear on a piece of paper hundreds of feet away.

"And what can your teacher do?" he asked the other disciple.

"My teacher can also perform amazing feats," the other student replied. "When he's tired, he sleeps. When hungry, he eats."

When your body signals to you and you answer appropriately, it is truly an amazing feat. Your thoughts, feelings, and cravings often stand in the way. Even Zen masters know how hard it is to respond to the body's needs.

In this chapter, you've taken a step closer to being able to thoughtfully and nonjudgmentally observe the clues that your body and thoughts send you. Through paying close attention to what is going on inside, you can respond to your hunger in a wise and conscious manner.

CHAPTER 6

being in the moment

*The secret of health for both mind and body is not to mourn
for the past, worry about the future, or anticipate troubles,
but to live in the present moment wisely and earnestly.*
—Buddha

Ella packed her lunch in a brown paper bag every day, and she would devour her lunch as she drove from school to work. Like many people, she was chronically overworked and stressed out. One day when she was running late for work, she stopped at a red light. She anxiously tapped her fingers on the steering wheel. Surely, she was going to be late, she thought. She looked over at the brown bag, remembering that she had packed leftover pizza. But the pizza was gone. For a moment, she wasn't sure what had happened to it. She wondered if she had actually put it in the bag. Then, she saw a little bit of tomato sauce on her hands, and she suddenly realized that she had already eaten it. She didn't even remember tasting one bite. She had been so worried about getting to her next destination that she did not even realize that she had switched to autopilot, as she did every day. Ella made a pact with herself to stop eating in the car.

The following chapter is meant to help you learn how to eat calmly in the present moment. It's likely that you often eat really good food, but you aren't really there to enjoy it. Like Ella did in her car, it's easy to let the mind wander. Ella's story is an extreme version of mindless eating. But this type of eating, on a smaller scale, often happens when you are so focused on the TV, for example, that you don't really realize that you are eating until the program ends. Or, perhaps you wander through the kitchen grabbing handfuls of chips or cookies without really being very aware of why.

In this chapter you'll learn how to be more present with your body, your emotions, and your experience of stress, and you'll be introduced to some strategies, including breathing and relaxation exercises, that will help you deal with emotions and stress. Being in the moment includes turning off your autopilot behaviors, being present as you eat, and not doing a hundred different things during meals. You will start to notice when you are engaged in a frantic quest to fill yourself up or to find something that will finally satisfy you, rather than enjoying what you have.

turn off autopilot

Being in the present moment is a tricky skill for most of us. We live a lot of our life on autopilot mode, in which we just go through the motions. Sometimes it is just easier to act out of habit and routine. Maybe going with the flow helps us to feel less overwhelmed by juggling so many responsibilities in one day.

The downside of acting on autopilot is that the enjoyment of whatever you are doing is sucked right out of it. Automatic actions leave you feeling numb and sometimes even empty. Think about what happens when you drive mindlessly; you might feel completely detached and numb. You miss the scenery. It's almost as if you've left your body. The experience is completely different from the exhilaration you may have felt when you first started driving. Think about how exciting it was to drive when you first got your driver's license. At that time, you noticed everything and looked at it through fresh eyes.

> ## Mindful Eating Tip: *Shifting Your Routine*
>
> When you struggle with mindlessness, it's highly likely that mindlessness appears in many areas of your life. Maybe you shift onto autopilot in your job; you've got your duties so down pat that you can think about a hundred other things while you're working. Or maybe you act mindlessly in your relationship. You know what to expect from your spouse to the point that you often don't even let him or her finish a sentence.
>
> By working on rearranging a few of your everyday routines, you may be able to cut down on some of your autopilot eating without much effort. For example, let's say you find yourself sitting on the couch and watching TV every night after work. It's like clockwork. You can't seem to work yourself out of this mindless habit. Instead of working on changing the eating routine, try shifting your other ingrained habits. For example, tape your favorite TV show and watch it at a different time. Or, if you find yourself getting caught up in night eating, try shifting the times you go to bed and get up.

Similarly, consider whether you really enjoy food when you are eating it while on autopilot mode, like mindlessly chomping on a bagel as you drive or grazing on a bowl of nuts as you watch TV. So many of my clients talk about feeling empty. Food is often something they turn to as a way to try to fill up that emptiness. Yet the way they are eating may be contributing to that sense of disconnection from their body. Taking a closer look at your entire life, not just the way you eat, might be a good start. Are you running from activity to activity? Are you just doing what you always do? It is harder to really be in the moment than it is to dwell on things you have to get done? Does this lead to a feeling of emptiness or hollowness inside?

We spend so much time dwelling on the past and anticipating the future that there is little time to enjoy life as it is right now. Consider for a moment what it would be like if you always rode a bike mindlessly. Imagine if you were constantly scanning a few blocks ahead or looking over your shoulder while riding that bike. Not only would it be complicated, it could be dangerous. You'd be very fortunate if you didn't get into an accident. So where is your mind when it's not in the moment? It's often sorting through many different thoughts.

When you eat mindfully, you start by just recognizing the tendency to be on automatic pilot. Say to yourself, "There I go again, I shifted into autopilot, just doing without thinking." After you are aware of the tendency, you make a commitment to yourself: commit to noticing the habit and placing your full attention in the moment. Intentionally direct your eyes toward your hand to watch it reaching for another cookie. Draw your attention to the fact that you are standing in front of the refrigerator. Ask yourself a very difficult question in that moment, "Do I really want this, or am I just following my old habits? If I were really sitting in the driver's seat rather than operating on autopilot, what direction would I go? Would I stop here? Or would I keep going?"

When you are in the moment, your mind notices things as they happen. Put aside the rest of the thoughts you are juggling while you eat, and make the task at hand your main priority. A significant culprit of autopilot behavior is multitasking.

stop multitasking

To eat mindfully, it's important to try to stop or limit multitasking while you eat. Too often we eat on the run. We eat in our cars and at our desks. You might find yourself eating at a breakneck speed or cramming in a meal while you work. Mindless eating is a symptom of the fast, treadmill-like pace of daily life.

According to research, dividing your attention between two tasks can actually interfere with mindful eating. Participants in a recent study listened to a detective story while they ate a meal. Those women who were distracted by the story ate 15 percent more (72 additional calories) and enjoyed their food less than those who were simply focused on their meal (Bellisle and Dalix 2001). Studies also show that eating while you drive causes more accidents than talking on your cell phone.

Multitasking while you eat makes eating seem like an unimportant task. It's interesting that people spend hundreds of thousands of dollars finding ways to improve their eating yet treat it as if it were a side task, not an important enough job to warrant giving it their complete attention.

Mindful eating is an opportunity to slow down. You reestablish the link between your brain and stomach. It doesn't mean you have to have long, leisurely meals complete with linen napkins and candlelight. It's about giving meals your complete attention, whether it be for five minutes or a half hour.

TV Trance

Do you get into a mindless eating trance the moment your TV is flipped on? Watching TV may be behind some of your mindless eating habits. Granted, watching TV isn't the only culprit of mindless eating. However, many studies continue to come back to the same thing (Gore et al. 2003): there is a significant correlation between how much TV you watch and how much you struggle with mindless overeating. Why? Following are a few reasons.

- TV time is replacing more active pursuits such as walking, riding your bike, or even doing housework.

- Watching TV is a sedentary activity. This leads to a decrease in your metabolic rate of burning calories. Resting or sleeping also causes a dip, but not as low as TV watching. Your body actually gets more benefit from doing nothing than from watching TV.

> ## Mindful Eating Tip: *Be Present*
>
> If your mind leaves, simply invite it to come back to the table. It hasn't been excused yet! You will be surprised at how much more conscious you are when you give eating 100 percent of your attention. If you want a snack, that is great—just stop what you are doing and be very present while you eat. Try turning off the TV and eliminating other distractions, like the radio, which tend to increase the likelihood of mindless eating.

- All programs, whether the news or a movie, have commercials, a lot of which are advertising unhealthy or junk foods. Repeatedly viewing these visual cues can stimulate your appetite even when you aren't hungry.

- TV is a distraction. It divides your attention between two tasks. You can't be totally tuned in to the process of eating when your eyes and mind are directed toward the screen.

- You may eat in rhythm with the TV. Sometimes people unconsciously continue to eat until the end of the program.

- TV watching may be a habit or a substitute for company. When you eat with other people, this can often keep your mind anchored in the moment.

You don't have the power to get rid of all the fast food joints or tempting foods that sometimes sabotage your mindful eating. However, cutting down on TV time when you eat is completely within your power.

mindful eating exercise: turning off distractions

If you consume snacks or meals in front of the TV, do an experiment: The next time you find yourself in front of the TV with a snack in hand, try turning off the TV. Eat your snack. Watch closely what happens inside. Does having the TV off change the way you would normally eat the snack? Does it seem uncomfortable? Sometimes people notice the silence. Others remark that they hear themselves chewing, something they didn't notice when covered up by a blaring TV. Do you notice a shift in how intentional you are about what you are eating? Try doing this exercise several times.

multitasking mindless eater

TV is just one of the many distractions that contribute to mindless eating. Complete the following questions to check in with yourself. Evaluate the many ways in which you might be caught multitasking while eating.

Ask yourself these questions. Answer yes or no.

_____ Do I eat while I drive?

_____ Do I stand in front of the refrigerator or in the pantry and eat?

_____ Do I graze on food?

_____ Do I eat while I am working at my desk?

_____ Do I eat while I watch TV?

_____ Do I eat and text message at the same time?

_____ Do I eat and read a book at the same time?

_____ Do I eat while listening to music?

_____ Do I eat while I am talking on the phone?

_____ Do I not even realize what I am eating because I am so distracted by something else?

_____ Do I eat while I am reading the newspaper?

_____ Do I snack while I am making dinner?

_____ Do I eat while I am talking to other people?

_____ Am I so busy that I feel as if I am always eating on the run?

---

body in the here and now!

Rachel, one of my clients, looked back at pictures of herself from five and ten years ago and said, "Look, I was so thin. Why didn't I appreciate what I looked like at the time? It's funny. I felt so fat even then. How could that be?" When those pictures were taken, Rachel felt just as bad about herself as she does now.

It is often difficult to feel satisfied with food or your life in the present moment. You have barely gotten comfortable where you are when you start looking to the next thing. You want more and more. Suddenly, the dream home you've been saving for after the starter home doesn't seem good enough. You are always looking for a better job, house, partner, and vacation. It's as if we are climbing the corporate life ladder. The same is true with your body and weight. Where you are never seems good enough. It's a rare skill to be able to stop and appreciate the present—or the present state of your body—before saying, "What next?"

Mindless Food Rules

People with eating issues often develop rules around food rather than listen to their hunger in the moment as it is happening. They allow the rules to dictate what they will and will not eat, rather than make a decision as it presents itself. Dieters, in particular, crave food rules. Because you have to eat three times a day, and because resisting the unhealthy foods can be so difficult, sometimes you want a system that makes it easy. It seems to be less effort to just have rules to follow than to think through each decision. Some examples of food rules might be the following: (1) no sugar, (2) no snacks after 8:00 P.M., and (3) no cream cheese (or only the fat-free version).

Ironically, rules sometimes increase mindless behavior. They don't take into consideration the context of the situation or your hunger level. So, when faced with a cake at a party (a no-no on your list of rules), you sigh in relief—you can just mindlessly follow your food rule. However, imagine that you are faced with a birthday cake, and it's your birthday cake. Now what do you do? You can't refuse a piece of your own birthday cake, but you don't want to break your rule. You may not even be consciously aware of what your food rules are. As you start to pay attention to your behaviors and thoughts, you may notice yourself explaining rules to yourself when you struggle with whether to eat something or pass it up.

What are your food rules? List them below.

_____

_____

_____

In this space, describe how you can make these rules more mindful. For example, for the rule, "I can't eat after 7:00 P.M.," a more mindful version would be, "I tend to avoid eating after 7:00 P.M. because I'm generally not hungry at that time (which means that if I were eating, then I would be doing so mindlessly). I will eat after 7:00 P.M. if I am really hungry, I missed dinner, or I'm in the mood for a mindful snack."

_____

_____

_____

Why do you lean on these rules?

_____

_____

When you buy a new car, you often look for the safest vehicle possible, with air bags and high safety ratings. Of course, if you are a reckless driver, the safest car in the world wouldn't keep you safe. People try to use food rules to keep them safe. They want the rules to protect them from mindless eating. If you feel this way, work on becoming a better driver of your eating habits instead. That would ultimately be the best approach to keep you out of harm's way.

Let's now take inventory of what you do have and want to appreciate about your body in this moment.

dear mindful body . . .

Write a letter to your body addressing the issue of acceptance. Tell your body what body parts have been easy to accept (for example, your legs, neck, and so on) and what parts have been hard to accept (for example, your stomach and thighs). Next, you'll write back as if your body is talking back to you. Discuss what your body would appreciate if you were able to accept it mindfully (stop trying to squeeze into tight clothes and have more energy with better foods). Remember, you don't have to love your body, but you do have to accept it as it is in this moment.

Dear Body,

_____

_____

_____

_____

_____

_____

_____

Sincerely,
   Mindful Self

Dear Mindful Self,

_____

_____

_____

_____

_____

_____

_____

Sincerely,
   Body

mindful eating exercise: practice being in the moment————

The mind becomes scattered when we try to escape the present moment. You might try to escape by trying to run away from unpleasant experiences (catching yourself eating mindlessly, pain, stress, and guilt), and by clinging to pleasant experiences (the taste of good food, and feeling in control, for example). It's easy to get upset about the unpleasant ("Darn, I'm eating mindlessly again! I can't believe it") and cling to the pleasant ("I don't want this feeling to stop!"). You might also evade the present by jumping ahead to the future ("Things will be better next month") or dwelling on the past ("I miss the way it was!"). When you notice your attention slipping away, look around you. Notice what is going on right now. Draw your attention to the way your chair feels against your legs. What do you hear around you? Notice how your feelings change when you focus in on what *is* happening right now rather than what *might* happen in the future or what *has* happened.

One way to draw your attention back into the moment and anchor yourself back to your body is to notice your jewelry, if you are wearing any. People are often so accustomed to the feeling of their wedding ring on their hand, for example, that they no longer feel it. Bring your attention to your ring or a necklace and notice how it feels against your skin. You will likely find that you have moved your awareness back into your body for a moment.

————

mindfulness of feelings

*I've noticed that there is usually something behind my mindless eating binges.
Sometimes, it is hard for me to put a finger on it. I do a mini self-check. Am I
hungry, lonely, or tired from work? It's typically one of the above. If none of these resonates,
it's likely to be just some really yummy food hanging around that has caught my eye.
Knowing my top triggers helps me to at least take a moment to pause. I am mindful of the
impulse and consciously draw my awareness to it.*
—Alexa

After a new client finishes telling me a story about a mindless-eating incident, I always ask the same question: "What were you feeling right before it happened?" The client will frequently scrunch her eyebrows together and reply, "I don't know what I was feeling" or "Nothing, I wasn't feeling anything." I remind clients that even feeling nothing is feeling something. Emptiness is an emotion. After a few sessions, my clients can anticipate that this question is coming. But, they are now ready with a response because they have learned to mindfully identify their feelings.

People are like vending machines. Push the right button and out comes a very predictable response. We can see it most clearly with emotions. For example, your spouse likely knows your "hot buttons," the things that can send you skyrocketing into anger in a second. We also have very predictable triggers of mindless eating. Many things trigger mindless eating: seeing a pizza commercial on TV, being around other people who are eating mindlessly, and the smell of fresh-baked pie. Emotions like stress and boredom can also be powerful automatic triggers. For this reason, it's important to become an expert on how you feel.

Here are a few reasons a person may be out of touch with his or her feelings. Read these over and see if any of these reasons might apply to you:

Mindfulness Tip: *The Lifeguard*

Think about your mind as if it were a lifeguard. Just sit back and observe the activity swimming around in your mind. But sometimes, when you realize that you are drowning in your thoughts, you need to jump in to rescue yourself. If so, read the sections in chapter 8 that focus on nonjudgmental thinking. Or, do the activity on mindless thinking in chapter 8 to try to prevent yourself from sinking any further into negative thoughts.

- The feeling did not start immediately before the mindless eating (for example, you were angry the day before and still feeling blah all the next day, rather than experiencing anger that suddenly started two minutes before you began eating).

- The feeling is subtle. (Intense negative and positive feelings are easier to notice than weak or complex emotions.)

- You are disconnected from your body and feelings.

- You don't have a clear sense of how the emotions and mindless eating are connected.

- You are moving too quickly to slow down and check in with how you feel.

- You are overwhelmed by conflicting emotions (for example, you love and hate your partner at the same time).

- You don't know how to put your feeling into words.

- Growing up, you didn't have a good role model for how to identify and process feelings.

- You stuff down or ignore your feelings, or you don't think feelings are important.

mindful exercise: putting feelings under a mindful microscope ———

Below are some basic steps that you can use to identify and process what you feel in relation to mindless eating. This exercise walks you through discovering and labeling the feeling and determining how it is expressed.

1. **Acknowledge:** First, recognize that a feeling is actually happening right here and right now. Say to yourself, "Oh yes, there it is. I am having a feeling." Ask yourself what event prompted this feeling. For example, "I feel angry at myself. It started when I mindlessly ate appetizers at a party." Write about your feeling and its trigger below:

   _____

   _____

   _____

2. **Describe:** Label emotions in the moment they happen: jealousy, happiness, excitement, irritation, anger, frustration, happiness, boredom. Be very specific about the emotion. Consider the subtle, but important, differences between "angry" and "enraged," for example. You become less entangled with the emotion when you can accurately and clearly identify the emotion. Imagine how misunderstood you would feel if someone believed you were hurt when you were actually angry. Say, "I am feeling _____."

   What kind of emotional range do you have? Do you have deep valleys and hills, or do you maintain a fairly even keel (a restricted range). Use at least three words to describe the feeling you are having ("I feel guilty, irritable, and angry with myself," for example):

   _____

   _____

3. **Allow:** Accepting how you feel does not mean rationalizing, condoning, or justifying the feelings. In other words, you don't have to like the feelings or even be okay with them. You are simply allowing emotions to be present, whatever the feelings are at that moment. You don't judge or censure your feelings. Nor do you downplay your emotions by thinking, "Other people have it worse than I do," or "I shouldn't feel that way." Say to yourself, "I can feel this without trying to change it or wishing it away."

   Why am I having difficulty accepting this feeling as it is? Describe any urges to change it. For example, you might say, "It makes me feel uncomfortable to feel angry and guilty for mindlessly eating. I get this urge to punish myself or to try to make it go away. Instead, I will just notice the anger."

4. **Explore the inside:** Emotions are complex events. They are a combination of bodily sensations, thoughts, feelings, motivations, and attitudes. Notice where and how you experience your feelings physically. Perhaps when you feel sad, you have a lot of aches and pains, or you become tired. Or maybe you are easily prone to colds, other viruses, and headaches during times of stress. Below, write how your emotions feel in your body, and how they come across in your thoughts. For example, "I feel the anger as heat. I become flushed. When I'm angry I tend to think about everything else in my life that makes me angry."

mindful eating exercise: mindfulness of emotions scale ─────

When you are mindful of your emotions, you allow yourself to experience them, no matter how good or bad they feel. The more aware you are of the intensity of your emotional reactions, the more familiar you will become with how you respond emotionally to certain food situations.

Start the process of understanding the range of your feelings by looking at the scale on the next page. Check in with your feelings several times a day. Use it to identify how you feel when you eat. But also use it to look at the emotions that come up during your daily routines.

Mindfulness of Emotions Scale

10   Deep, intense feelings, like disgusted, depressed, ashamed, anxious. Desire to punish self for "bad" behavior. Feel undeserving. Running from feelings. Continually wishing bad feelings would go away.

9   Very unpleasant emotions, such as awful and guilty. Mostly consumed by negative feelings.

8   Moderately uncomfortable. Fairly critical. Somewhat guilty. A nagging feeling that maybe you shouldn't eat that. Very distasteful emotions emerging that are difficult to let go of.

7   Slight concern. A little regretful. Some distress and uneasiness.

6   A dab of discomfort. Negative emotions are fleeting.

5   Neutral feelings. Not positive or negative. Food just is what it is. It isn't good or bad. People often experience neutral feelings when eating fruits or vegetables. When mindful, you strive to maintain a sense of neutrality.

4   Mildly positive emotions. Pretty good. Content.

3   Pleased. Happy. Relaxed. As if you had a small treat.

2   Extreme pleasure. Joyful, excited, blissful.

1   On a high. Cloud nine. Ecstatic. Clinging to positive feelings. Not wanting feelings to end.

---

mindful emotions

Some Eastern religions include the notion of the "hungry ghosts." They live in the underworld and are depicted as teardrop shaped, with big, bloated stomachs. They are constantly craving food (sound familiar)? Yet, these hungry ghosts have necks that are too thin to pass food. As a result, eating is incredibly painful for them. Some of the ghosts are described as having mouths the size of a needle's eye and stomachs the size of a mountain. The ghosts are a metaphor. They represent people's inability to make themselves feel better by fulfillg their physical urges and desires. Food just doesn't make us feel better in the long term.

We are all very much like the hungry ghosts. At times the desire for food is enormous, but even when you eat, you don't feel satisfied—emotionally satisfied. Feelings like jealousy, longing, loneliness, and sadness continue to haunt you whether you eat or not.

Have you ever wondered why some people overeat when they are depressed? Food naturally increases neurotransmitters, particularly your serotonin level, which is a chemical in the brain that is responsible for alleviating depression. Other healthy behaviors, like exercising or talking to friends, can also raise serotonin levels. But people frequently lean too heavily on eating to lift their moods. Other coping behaviors, when you are able to use them, often provide longer-lasting benefits.

A common misperception is that only negative emotions spark mindless eating. In fact, it is quite the contrary. Negative *and* positive feelings urge people to eat. Eating tasty foods makes people happy. We often want to hang onto that feeling of happiness in any way possible.

Mindful Eating Tip: *Observing Feelings from a Distance*

To step out of your feelings, try the following:

Instead of saying:	"I'm worried about calories."
	"I'm angry at myself for overeating."
	"I'm afraid of losing control."
	"I can't stand this guilt."
Add the word "the":	"The anger I'm experiencing regarding overeating is difficult."
	"The fear I'm noticing in myself is intense."
	"The guilt is haunting me."
	"I'm having thoughts that lead me to worry about calories."
	"I'm having the *feeling* of anger at myself for overeating."
	"I'm having the *thought* of guilt."

This new language helps you to remember that what is going on inside is just a thought or a feeling. It doesn't have complete power over you.

---

your hungry ghosts (or feelings)

Positive feelings that prompt mindless eating. Provide some examples below ("M&Ms in the afternoon at work tasted so good. They were a bright spot in my day, and I didn't want it to end," for instance).

_____

_____

Negative feelings that prompt mindless eating. Make a list of feelings that are tough to handle, the emotions that prompt you to engage in mindless eating. Notice how your emotions change when you eat (for example, eating pushes away uncomfortable feelings, numbs them, or covers them up).

_____

_____

_____

_____

mindful stress management

When I'm stressed out, I will eat everything that isn't nailed down in the house.
—Nancy

You cannot manage your weight without using solid stress management techniques. It's nearly impossible. A large body of research has been focused on the connection between stress hormones and weight gain and loss, and researchers have found that, in some people, stress can make weight cling to the body.

According to a recent study published in *Natural Medicine* (Warne and Dallman 2007), mice under chronic stress became obese compared to non-stressed mice fed the same high-fat, high-sugar diet. The researchers asserted that it is likely caused by a combination between the diet and stress level.

your stressors

What are your top three stressors; both positive and negative? (An example of a positive stressor might be the process of planning a wedding; it's a good thing, but it certainly can cause a lot of stress. An example of a negative stressor might be receiving too many unreasonable demands at work.)

1. _____

2. _____

3. _____

What are your healthy coping mechanisms?

_____

What are your unhealthy coping mechanisms?

_____

Putting It into Perspective

Think of the most stressful event or situation you have experienced. How does the current stress relate to that incident? Is it more or less stressful?

_____

_____

_____

_____

How did you cope with the previous stressor? If that coping mechanism was helpful, could you take a similar approach in this circumstance? For example, perhaps you gained support from family members to help you cope with an illness. Could you use this same strategy to gain support now?

_____

_____

_____

_____

_____

Unfortunately, you cannot get rid off all the stress in your life; it isn't possible. You probably wouldn't want it all to go away. A little bit of stress adds some excitement and drama to our lives. Without it, life would be kind of boring. Besides, certain events that are stressful are also positive, like planning moving into a new home. It's when you don't think you can cope with it that stress becomes negative.

stress-check worksheet

Signs of Stress

How do you know when you are stressed out? In the worksheet below, put a check mark next to any of the statements that apply to you.

_____ I'm feeling overwhelmed.

_____ I don't know where to start.

_____ I'm feeling a little anxious.

_____ I have physical symptoms such as tense muscles and headache.

_____ I find myself procrastinating.

_____ I'm experiencing stomach problems.

_____ I have trouble falling asleep, or I lie awake thinking.

_____ I'm worrying.

_____ I have high blood pressure.

_____ I've had a change in appetite (either a loss of appetite or increase in stress eating).

_____ I've been taking medication such as aspirin for headache or aches and pains.

Where do you experience stress the most? For example, does stress show itself most in your thoughts (guilt and worry), emotions (anxiety, depression), or body (headaches, tension)?

If you start to feel any of the above symptoms, it is time for an immediate action plan to mindfully deal with the stress. This means *responding* (with a planned action) rather than *reacting* (with automatic ways of coping) to stressful events and feelings.

Your Level of Stress

Sometimes you can get more perspective about your problems when you figure out just how severe your stress is. On a scale of 1 to 10, how would you rate your level of stress?

Has the level increased or decreased in the past day, week, or month?

Annoying or Life Changing?

Just how significant is this stressor? Sometimes people react to little stressors as if they were major, life-changing events. Ask yourself, "How important is this situation? Is it simply annoying, frustrating, and difficult to deal with? Or is it a life-or-death situation? Could this situation change my life drastically? Will it alter its course just a little? Or will it probably not affect it at all?

Try to put your stress into perspective. In this space, write about the true level of importance of this stressful event in your life:

Mindful Stress Management Techniques

Here are a few techniques you can try when you are feeling stressed:

- **Do a brief stress check.** Fill out the worksheets on the two previous pages. Then ask yourself, "Am I thinking about this stress in a way that helps or hurts the situation?"

    The greatest weapon against stress is our ability to choose one thought over another.
    —William James

- **Reduce the *physiological* aspects of stress.** The physical effects of stress do a lot of damage to your body; 60 to 90 percent of doctor visits are due to stress-related illnesses. You may not be able to eliminate the stressful event. But you are able to manage how much stress is expressed through your body. Try a breathing exercise (see page 121) to help to move your body out of stress mode into a state of relaxation. You will be much better able to handle the stress if your body is calm.

    It's not stress that kills us, it is our reaction to it.
    —Hans Selye

- **Set a time to mindfully worry.** If you can't put the stressful event aside, and you find yourself unable to stop worrying, be mindful about your worry. Set a mindfulness clock (see the Online Resources section) or set a timer. Allow yourself to just focus on the worry and nothing else during that time. When the alarm goes off, stop what you are doing and devote all of your attention to the worry thoughts; this is an alternative to trying to worry about it while you are doing other things.

- **Download mindfulness meditations.** Try the guided body scans, meditations, or CDs available for download or purchase on the sites listed in the Online Resources section. Check out relaxation tapes from the library. Or create a playlist of relaxing music to download to your mp3 player.

Secret Benefits of Deep Breathing

Are you skeptical about whether breathing exercises work? If so, you're not alone. My clients often say, "I breathe all day long. How is this really going to help?" The breathing in this exercise is a special kind. It is simply intended to relax your body and bring your mind back into the present moment so you can be more aware. The good news is that the exercise only takes seconds.

Mindful breathing comes with benefits that might surprise you:

- **Weight management.** Yes, it's true! Improving your breathing will help you deal with emotional issues that lead to food cravings and food fears. When you are calm, you are less likely to turn to food for comfort. Also, the additional oxygen you get from mindful breathing allows the body to digest food properly, which helps with weight management.

- **Increased energy.** Are you always tired? Breathing increases energy by boosting oxygen levels in your bloodstream, the opposite of holding your breath, which many people do when they are anxious. Deep breathing helps retrain your body to take in more oxygen. When you have more energy, your awareness is open, and you are ready to tackle the challenge of mindful eating.

> ### Mindful Eating Tip: *Anchor to This Very Moment*
> Think of breathing as an anchor. Deep, mindful breaths help to anchor your mind and feelings when you feel as if you are starting to drift away or are being swept away by a current of emotions.

- **Clearer thinking.** Increasing oxygen to the brain actually allows you to slow down, focus your thoughts, and respond to events more clearly, rationally, and calmly.

- **Reduced stress.** Deep breathing is the easiest way to work through stress. You can do breathing exercises anywhere and in response to any stressful event. If you begin to breathe slowly, you can trick your body into thinking it is moving into a state of relaxation. Think about what your breathing is like when you are about to fall asleep. That's the type of breathing that will help you reduce stress.

- **Body boost.** When you actively improve your breathing, you can change involuntary activities of your sympathetic nervous system, which regulates blood pressure, heart rate, circulation, digestion, and many other bodily functions. Studies show that people who use deep breathing can actively slow down the heart rate and brain waves in the area of the brain that controls emotion.

one minute stress reducer: mindful belly breathing

Try this mindful belly breathing technique at least once a day or whenever you find your mind dwelling on upsetting thoughts. (You can also simply take a slow, deep breath whenever you are experiencing difficulty with eating mindfully.)

First, do a self-check. How are you breathing now? Observe yourself. Are you breathing fast or slow? Are you having trouble breathing or none at all?

Next, try a deep breathing exercise. You can either stand up or lie down, whichever is most comfortable for you.

1. Find a comfortable place where you will not be disturbed. Turn off the phone and the TV.

2. Position yourself so you are comfortable.

3. Place one hand on your stomach.

4. Inhale slowly and deeply through your nose, starting at the bottom of your abdomen. Count slowly to three as you inhale.

5. Imagine your stomach expanding like a balloon being blown up.

6. Do a self-check. If you're breathing from your diaphragm, your hand will rise and you'll see your lower abdomen moving downward and outward.

7. Pause for a count of two.

8. Exhale slowly through your nose to a count of three.

9. Once you get the hang of the exercise, you may want to add another step. For example, you may want to say to yourself the word "mindful" or "relax" as you breathe in, and "mindless" or "stress" with each breath out. Inhale as you say the feeling or emotion you want to bring in. Exhale to release any stressful things you would like to let go of.

---

be here

Now that you have learned more about how to be in the moment, you will bring more awareness to your everyday meals. You may find that you can't always live in the moment. It's tough to be totally present at all times without thinking about what you are doing next. But as you practice and become more familiar with being in the moment, it can become an integral part of your life.

When you eat in the moment, you find yourself making decisions as they happen, and you find yourself rethinking your decisions after the fact less and less.

CHAPTER 7

‿‿‿‿ ‿‿‿‿ ‿‿‿‿ ‿‿‿‿ ‿‿‿‿ ‿‿‿‿ ‿‿‿‿ ‿‿‿‿ ‿‿‿‿ ‿‿‿‿

a mindful environment

Every being is the author of his own health or disease.
—Buddha

Jill, a twenty-nine-year-old woman, brought to her counseling session an advertisement that she had ripped off the wall of an elevator in her apartment building. Jill saw many ads there every day, but this particular ad drew her attention every time she stepped in the elevator. It was an image of a stick-thin nude model in a bathtub full of liquid chocolate, submerged as if it were a bubble bath.

On the surface, this was just an ad meant to sucker you into buying chocolate. But to Jill, it contained a much more disturbing message. The ad implied that you should forget about soaking in a nice bubble bath in order to relax. Instead, eat chocolate. But don't worry, you can still be unrealistically thin.

To a mindless eater, ads like this are toxic. They creep into the person's subconscious, like subliminal messages. Food makers do this because they are heavily invested in keeping mindless eating in business. Without mindless eaters in the world, they lose a lot of money. What better way to make money than to get mindless eaters to buy into the idea of using food to melt away the stress of the day while believing that they can still be thin. This is simply dangerous!

Jill was smart. She could spot an ad that promoted mindless eating a mile away, and ads like this caused a whirlwind of emotions to start inside her. She'd try to exercise as much self-restraint as possible, repeating to herself, "Chocolate is such a diet no-no. If I eat it, I'll have blown my diet again." At the same time, her mind raced with desire. "I love chocolate. I do feel good when I eat it. I really want some!"

Like most people, Jill found that her surroundings had the power to erode mindful eating habits. After weeks of this emotional tug-of-war, she simply tore down the advertisement. This solved one part of the problem. Some things in her environment, like this ad, she could control by simply taking it down. Other things she couldn't control, like the very same ad on a giant billboard along the highway.

Jill found a way to respond mindfully. She started noticing other things that triggered a desire for mindless eating, like TV commercials for pizza and coupons for fast food. When she experienced a craving, she would pay attention to it, but she was able to consciously decide what to do with it rather than let a subconscious war with her appetite take place.

Throughout this chapter, you will train your mind to look closely at your external environment. Your main task is to draw your awareness to your surroundings to see if they are a key player in sabotaging mindful eating. You'll investigate how your access to food affects the way you eat, the way images and messages in the media stimulate your appetite, and how what you say, to yourself and others, promotes or discourages mindless eating. We'll start out with a trip around your kitchen.

toxic environment

Our ancient ancestors must have wished they had the problem we face today: being inundated with too much food, much more than we could ever eat. Food is everywhere. We see it on fast-food billboards along highways, on advertisements for pizza on the back of bus benches, in vending machines in airports, and even in candy machines in bathrooms. TV commercials advertise foods that will help you to feel good and, even more important, "full." Try to relax by flipping through a magazine and you'll find that it is filled with pages of delicious desserts and fried-chicken recipes. In that same magazine, you will read about different diets that advise how to avoid eating so many calories. You will also see images of perfect bodies in skimpy bathing suits.

As you can see, we live in an environment that doesn't teach us many useful things about mindful eating. In fact, it is quite the opposite. Our culture gives us the message that we should be eating all the time. It also tells us that we should be dieting around the clock as well.

Given this type of culture, you have to work really hard to take control of what you can. This means setting up environments within your home and work space that help you, to the best of your ability, eat in a mindful way, or at least be aware of how the environment triggers your unconscious eating.

What Is a Mindful Eating Environment?

Think for a moment about whether you have a mindful eating environment. An important step in your mindful eating journey is to create mindful surroundings: a place to eat that is free from distraction (away from things like the TV, radio, work, and other distracters), is comfortable (a place where you can sit down in front of a table), and promotes mindful eating (fewer trigger foods).

Much of mindless eating has nothing to do with hunger. Instead, you are simply reacting to the cues in your environment. Let's say you are walking in the store and see a display advertising a two-for-one deal on corn chips. It's sitting right in the middle of the aisle. It's almost difficult to maneuver your cart around it. You say to yourself that maybe you could put these in your kid's lunch, so you throw the bags in the cart. When you get home, you place them at the very front of the cupboard. The bags are the first thing you see when you open the cabinet door. These corn chips have just become a booby trap for mindless eating. In part, this is because you have them in your home. But the biggest problem is that you have two large bags rather than one. The more you have, the less you will carefully think about what to do with it. Cheap food often prompts mindless eating because we have more of it.

Have you ever been offered a very small portion of something good, like the last corner of an expensive chocolate bar? When you have just a little of something, you often want to make it last. You might even ration the chocolate to yourself, eating only a little bit at a time, saving some for later. If you have a larger bag of cheap chocolate, your psychological approach to it is quite different. You are much more reckless about the way you eat it, with little concern for the need to savor it.

Again, how much food you surround yourself with at home is very important. I don't mean to suggest that you should completely get rid of all tempting food. However, the quantity is something many of us can work on. Think of it like this: if fish were swimming around in a bowl of clean water with just a sprinkle of food, the quality of the water would help to keep them healthy. But, if you threw in too much food, they'd struggle to survive. Why? Fish are very sensitive to overfeeding. Too much food in their environment begins to rot and becomes toxic to them. We are very similar to fish. When you have too much food in your environment, it becomes toxic to you. It's hard to remain healthy when the environment is saturated with food.

the mindful pantry

Consider whether you need to clean out your pantry or refrigerator. Go to your cupboard right now. Pick the shelf that contains the most food or the cupboard you use the most frequently. Carefully check out what type and how much food you own at this very moment. How would you describe your stash? Is it like a buffet on a cruise ship, with a wide variety of everything you like? Is it deserted, with few options? Is it jammed full of food that you bought a long time ago with the good intention of using but just haven't gotten around to yet? Is it full of healthy foods? Is it mostly ingredients for cooking with? Or is it a stock of prepared snack foods? The intention of this exercise is not to make you judge your choices but to help you understand what you are working with. Answer the questions below to help you consider your immediate environment.

Do I Have a Mindful Eating Environment?

_____ Do I keep foods that trigger significant mindless eating nearby or in easy access in my car, desk, or cupboards at home?

_____ Do I buy a variety of foods, including fruits, vegetables, and proteins?

_____ Do I buy foods that I know will trigger other people's mindless eating?

_____ Do I create a pleasant place to eat that is free from distractions—away from the TV and newspapers?

_____ Do I sit down when I eat?

_____ Do I eat at a table?

_____ Do I avoid eating when I work, talk on the phone, drive, and so on?

_____ Do I keep healthy foods in an easily accessible and visible place?

_____ Do I eat at fast-food restaurants?

How does the type of food you own right now influence your mindless and mindful eating? Say, for example, you buy things in bulk. Perhaps the big boxes encourage your mindless eating, because once they are open it is hard for you not to worry about the contents going to waste.

What do you imagine a more mindful cupboard or refrigerator would look like to you? Remember that it doesn't have to contain only fruits and vegetables. But maybe it would contain more choices, or perhaps you need fewer options? Too many choices may make it hard for you to pick.

Location, Location, Location

Mike, a forty-year-old welder, loves doughnuts. One day, when he came home from work, he walked into his kitchen and noticed a box of doughnuts that his wife had bought from his favorite doughnut shop. He sat down in front of the TV. For the next hour, all Mike could think about was the doughnuts. He tried to fight the urge. Instead, he ate the entire box.

The next day, he walked into the kitchen again when he got home from work. He didn't know it, but his wife had bought another box of doughnuts and put them in the cupboard. After an hour of watching TV, he headed toward the kitchen. When he opened up the cupboard, he was surprised to find more doughnuts. He ate two, rather than the whole box, this time. In this second situation, he was better able to refrain from mindless eating, perhaps because he didn't spend an hour

> ### Mindful Environment Tip:
> ### *Strategically Place Food*
>
> Studies show that where you keep food can dramatically impact your mindful and mindless eating habits. Foods kept in plain view are much more likely to be eaten mindlessly than those kept out of sight. Simply putting food away helps you to cut out a portion of mindless eating. The reverse is true as well. Keeping healthy foods handy, accessible, and in sight—for instance, in a bowl on the counter—will increase the likelihood that you will eat them. Remember, one of the reasons we love fast food is the convenience factor.

thinking about the doughnuts. Rather, they were only on his mind for a few minutes. Mike realized that it was okay to have these kinds of foods, but having them in plain view made it hard for him to stay mindful.

Mindless Trigger Foods

As we've discussed earlier in this book, a "trigger food" is one that is likely to initiate mindless eating: ice cream, fried chicken, or an oversized box of cookies. If trigger foods reliably lead to mindless eating, how do they find their way into our pantries? Some parents say things like, "I keep the chips because the kids like them" or "My spouse eats them." It's fine to have some mindless foods in the home. However, people often have too many of them, and they set up a mindless eating trap when you are just starting to rework your habits. You have to be honest about why you have them. Mostly, it's because they taste good.

The overall goal is to be able to have the foods you love and crave in your cupboard and be able to eat them in a mindful way, to savor and eat a sensible portion.

With certain trigger foods, such as sugary cereals and ice cream, it can take a very long time to learn to eat them in moderate portions. If this is the case for you, it may be better to cut these foods out for a while and start with more neutral foods like pretzels—foods that taste good to you but don't cause emotional turmoil.

When people first start trying to eat more mindfully, they often find it helpful to keep just one food in the home that they really love, an apple turnover, for example. (Do not get rid of all the foods you love; this is a setup for feeling deprived.) Put it in the freezer. Get it out to practice your mindful eating skills. When you've got the hang of eating the apple turnover, try a different item that you crave. Get the hang of the more neutral foods before trying the difficult trigger foods. This will help to raise your confidence.

People who undereat may have a different challenge. They may need to stock their shelves with a variety of healthy foods rather than keeping a small selection of diet foods. Having a stockpile of nonfat muffins and fat-free granola bars around may prompt you to stay in the deprived, diet mentality. You need a variety of healthy, whole foods.

A Mindful Table

Don't underestimate the importance of *where* you eat. Consider the difference between dining at a doughnut shop versus a sushi restaurant. Restaurants, in general, are often a hot spot for mindless eating. Or perhaps you find it difficult to eat mindfully at work.

A group of nurses made a simple change to their work space that significantly cut down on their collective mindless eating. They would keep treats and goodies that had been brought in by clients within arm's reach of the centrally located triage desk, which the nurses passed frequently all day long. Each time they passed, the nurses would take a handful of nuts or a nibble of a cookie. But a little bit here and a little bit there added up. When they realized this, they took a vote and decided to simply move the location of their snacks. Notice that they didn't get rid of the treats completely. Instead of putting them in the central location, they put all the snacks in the break room, which happened to be down a flight of stairs. This dramatically cut down on their daily mindless eating. To get a snack, they had to make a special effort to get it. Because of their limited time and busy work schedules, getting to the break room happened once a day rather than all day long. In addition, they got a little extra exercise going up and down the stairs.

One of the nurses took this strategy to her home. She kept a bag of cookies in her linen closet on the second floor of her home. She didn't do this to hide it. She gave herself total permission to have them. But putting them in a more distant location made her more conscious of her eating. When she was home during the day, she noticed that she only went to get a cookie when she really, really wanted one, rather than taking a nibble because they just happened to be in the kitchen.

Julie, a client, spoke about keeping her husband's candy and snacks in his own separate drawer. She considered these to be "his food" that she wasn't supposed to touch because she was on a diet. But, like clockwork, every time she passed the drawer when she was home alone, she would open it. Just having a no-no drawer like this was a setup. So, she asked her husband to move his candy stash to his office, and she filled the drawer with nonfood items. She considered replacing the candy with healthy snacks. However, the drawer had become so associated with mindless eating that she was afraid that she would even overeat the healthy snacks.

Another client, Miranda, discussed feeling good about her at-home eating habits, but she struggled to eat mindfully at dinner parties. She always seemed to throw in the towel when she was out of her home element. She realized that she was really influenced by how much those around her ate. She didn't want people to think she was rude or didn't like the food if she ate less. To change this, she learned to approach dinner parties with a different mind-set, although it took time for her to learn to worry less about what other people thought about her actions and begin to focus more on her mindful eating.

Getting a good handle on the environments that trigger mindless eating is key. The more aware you are of the type of environment that is a mindless-eating trap door, the more you can find ways to step around the trap door.

mindful locations

Carefully think through where the majority of your mindful and mindless eating takes place, and write your thoughts below:

_____

_____

_____

_____

Consider the environments where you are most vulnerable (for example, at work, around the refrigerator, while watching TV, in restaurants). Write your thoughts below:

_____

_____

_____

_____

Write about the environments that are most helpful (for example, eating with healthy friends, sitting down at your table, eating in the morning):

_____

_____

_____

_____

Use the list above to help you thoughtfully approach these settings. When you are in vulnerable situations, you will need to be particularly diligent with your mindful eating skills. Sometimes you might even want to steer clear of these locations. And at times you will be able to; if it is a particular restaurant that prompts you to mindlessly eat, you can find another restaurant option. But sometimes you can't avoid these places. If that is the case, your task is to understand what it is about these particular environments that facilitates mindless overeating. You may need to get creative and think of ways to make it a better place to eat.

Keep in mind that there are some places where you do eat more mindfully. You can't forget or ignore this. Think about what it is about these environments that facilitates mindful eating. Use this information to help rearrange other settings, and consider eating there more often.

If you feel as if you struggle with mindless eating everywhere you go, and there don't seem to be any situations that help you eat in a mindful way, don't panic. This just means you feel extremely overwhelmed by the mindless eating environment around you. It's no surprise, since we come across food constantly. You may want to pick just one place to start working on your mindless eating. Choose a setting that is fairly easy to start with, rather than beginning with the most challenging one. Just focus your efforts on making one place more mindful. Make it comfortable, free from distractions and free from trigger foods.

shopping mindfully

Mindful eating really begins at the grocery store. Buying foods that promote mindful eating is half the battle. For this reason, it is extremely important to mindfully approach the way you shop. The good news is that this book will help you learn how to bring all of your mindful eating skills to the store with you.

Maya, one of my clients, revealed the dread she felt when going to the grocery store before she attended the mindful eating support group. After a time, she was able to apply her new mindful eating skills as she walked through the store. First, she took note of the times she felt a strong pull to put particular foods, like a sugary cereal or package of sweet buns, in her cart. Each time she felt that pull, she would check in with herself about why she wanted it. Was it the advertising on the package pulling her in? Was it a food she bought every week out of routine? Was it a food that was one of her top mindless-eating triggers?

Instead of letting her urges control the shopping trip, she went armed with a specific list that she had drawn up ahead of time. This significantly cut down on her impulse buys, and it also reduced her purchases of the foods she promised herself she would only eat in small portions but knew she couldn't. She walked through the store compassionately acknowledging her cravings and sticking to the list she had mindfully made at home.

The person in your home who does the grocery shopping has an enormous amount of power. He or she controls a significant portion of what goes into the mouths of the entire family. Consider what a huge responsibility that is! According to Brian Wansink, Director of the Cornell University Food and Brand Lab, a significant portion of our food purchases are unplanned and prompted by creative marketing tactics to urge you to impulsively buy more. We buy a lot of what we don't need, particularly foods that encourage mindless eating, because of tricky marketing techniques. (See www.foodpsychology.cornell.edu for more information on the way advertising suckers us into mindless shopping and eating. It provides an eye-opening look at why you spend so much money at the grocery store, even when you only went in for one item.)

What Is Mindful Shopping?

Mindful shopping means turning your awareness on full throttle when you go to the store. You are conscious of your thoughts and cravings, and you do not judge yourself for them, nor do you give in to them without thinking.

Consider whether your subconscious pushes the cart. A mindless mind responds automatically to flashy food displays, pictures of frozen cheesecakes and nachos (or foods that are "safe" and low fat if you are a dieter). You might also go into autopilot mode, buying the same things over and over again. Some people find that they are better able to keep their awareness focused and on target if they have a plan. Making a list can really help keep you in the moment rather than swept away by urges and cravings.

It's difficult to shop when you are the only person in your family who seems to worry about what you eat. Clients often say, "It's not fair. My husband can eat whatever he wants" or "My other family members (or roommates) have no problem with food." They feel torn between making mindful choices at the grocery store and picking up items that their family would want them to buy. It's important to focus on yourself and your own journey. Do not get caught in the debate about how you think things should be. Think acceptance.

In addition, it's worth your while to set a positive example for your loved ones, especially if you are a parent of small children or teens. Even if your significant other, children, or roommates don't have weight issues, it doesn't mean that what they eat is healthy for their body.

Tips for Mindful Shopping

- Try a trip to the store in which you just observe your behavior. What is your buying strategy? Do you put food in your cart on impulse? Do you have a strict plan? Do you plan your meals as you go? Do you buy the cheapest items? Investigate how your shopping habits do or do not contribute to mindless eating.

- It's helpful to buy more real or whole foods rather than items that resemble food or are a version of it. For example, instead of buying cheese spread, buy real cheese. (You may have to look for the real foods, since the processed foods are often in the middle of the aisle and the real ones are on the fringe.) You'll find this strategy beneficial, since our bodies are wired to respond most effectively to unprocessed foods. You may notice that you have much less of an emotional reaction to apples than to a bag of processed apple chips. For a great description of why this is a helpful strategy, read *In Defense of Food: An Eater's Manifesto* by Michael Pollan.

- Avoid "deals" on multiple items unless you have a large family. These marketing ploys often clutter up your environment with mindless food. So you then have too much food in the home (three boxes rather than one) or giant boxes of food from wholesale clubs.

questions to consider about mindful shopping

Answer the following questions about your interactions with food:

Do you actively participate in cooking meals, buying food, and making meal choices? If so, that is great. Is there a way you could shop more mindfully?

_____

_____

_____

If not, what do you need to do to create a more mindful environment for yourself or your family? How can you be more active in mindfully cooking meals and buying food?

_____

_____

_____

Do you make a list? What is typically on your list?

_____

_____

_____

During your next shopping trip, what would make it a more mindful experience (for example, going shopping when you are not hungry, taking time to shop carefully rather than rushing through the store, making it a priority to try new items, or buying what would help your body rather than what looks appealing at that moment)?

_____

_____

_____

_____

For Parents:

Your children watch the *way* you eat. They listen to what you *say* about food. You might notice that they start to think about food in the same way you do. As toddlers, they will grab food right out of your hand. They soak up your eating habits like a sponge. And, although they may eat well now, it is inevitable that they will emulate your eating habits eventually.

If you have children, ask yourself, "Do I create a mindful eating environment for my kids?"

_____

_____

In ten years, if your children ate as they do now (or the way you do), are they likely to have an eating problem?

_____

_____

mindfully eating "green"

I don't mean eating your leafy greens. I'm talking about choosing foods that are healthy for you, your loved ones, and the environment. For those who have a hard time eating mindfully for themselves, sometimes it is helpful to think about the environmental impact of their food choices.

Sadly, I have many clients who don't believe themselves to be worth the effort. When they decide to make a change, they are often motivated by wanting to do something good for someone else. Many moms want to lose weight, and the thing that keeps them focused is their kids; they want to be able to be more physically active and play with their children. Or, they are afraid that something will happen to their health and their ability to care for their kids. Eventually, as they get the ball rolling, they start eating well for themselves and make their own lives a priority. Doing it for their kids is a bonus.

So what if you don't have kids, or the people around you don't inspire you to get motivated? You may want to eat mindfully for yourself and

Mindful Eating Tip: *Start Eating Green*

In 2007, the producers of the *Oxford English Dictionary* picked *locavore* as the best new word of the year. A locavore is someone who buys locally grown ingredients and food products. The food comes right from local farmers' markets or is grown in one's own garden. Locally grown products often taste better and are generally fresher and healthier, and they are better for the planet because they don't have to be transported by carbon-producing, gas-guzzling trucks over long distances. Buying products grown within a one-hundred-mile radius also saves on fuel costs; as a result, these products may cost less, and the money you pay for them goes directly into the local economy. Buying fresh fruits and vegetables grown locally is one step you can take to help create a mindful eating environment for yourself and the world.

for the health of the planet. Consider this one example. On average, it takes approximately twenty-five hundred gallons of water to produce a single pound of meat. So by eating mindfully, you might be able to have a positive effect on the world. I am not aiming to make you feel guilty. On the contrary, I am encouraging you to make eating mindfully your contribution to improving the landscape of the world.

Eradicate Doughnuts?

The good news is that there has been some great improvement over the past few years in reducing the societal factors that contribute to mindless eating. For example, trans-fatty acids, a harmful substance to the body, has been banned in many restaurants. Many food makers have followed suit by also getting rid of these toxic "trans fats."

In our society, there has also developed a much greater focus on promoting a healthy lifestyle for families, and a national concern about the health of our children. Attention is being drawn to the growing occurrence of childhood obesity. As a result, more people and organizations have begun to push for healthier school lunches, improve the content of children's meals in restaurants, and educate parents on what to feed their families. This is a mindful step in the right direction for our society.

The bad news is that many people may go too far when they are cleansing their environments of foods that trigger mindless eating. For example, a senior center on the East Coast stopped offering free doughnuts to its members, believing that these doughnuts could harm the health of the seniors. The seniors protested the removal of the doughnuts, since many of them wanted the choice to eat the doughnuts rather than have the issue decided for them. Also, cupcakes and cookies have become a controversial topic in schools. Some schools have banned them as a birthday or holiday treat, requiring parents to bring in only healthier snacks of fruits and vegetables.

It would be helpful to live in a world that promotes, educates, and teaches its citizens about mindful eating. However, we have to be cautious not to take away the right to enjoy tasty foods in moderation.

The media contribute a great deal to our confusion over what to eat and what not to eat, what's enough and what's too much. Let's take a look at how the media influence our food choices.

minding the media

A local burger joint placed fliers on the windshields of cars around my neighborhood. They were advertising two double-bacon cheeseburgers for the price of one. It just so happened I was starving that day. As soon as I spied the flier sitting on my window, I made a mad dash to the burger place. I inhaled my two burgers. I don't think my tongue even got a change to touch them. I hated myself for walking right into that one. I wish I had thrown the flier away. I know I would have made a better choice if I hadn't mindlessly reacted to the ad.
—Jack

My clients are often very hard on themselves for mindless eating, saying things like "I'm such an idiot! Why can't I just eat mindfully?" I always tell them that they have to give themselves a break. It is extremely difficult for even the most mindful person to eat consciously in our culture.

When people become mindful eaters, they pay attention to the many triggers around them, including advertising. Every day, you see hundreds of ads. You see them so often and in so many places that they often escape your awareness. You become habituated to them. Mindful eaters realize that the media is always trying to hook them into being a mindless eater. It's of great advantage to the advertisers: get this person suckered into a habit and we'll sell more!

media triggers of mindless overeating worksheet ———————

Ask yourself if you are vulnerable to the following triggers. Put a check mark next to the situations that apply to you.

_____ Advertisements for "good deals" (for example, two sandwiches for the price of one deal, or ninety-nine cents for a burger)

_____ Advertisements that encourage you to reward yourself with food (using phrases like "Indulge yourself," "You deserve it," or "You're worth it")

_____ Visual images of food (such as close-ups of mouthwatering foods and magazine-cover photos of luscious desserts)

_____ Advertisements suggesting that food is a good way to deal with emotions (showing comfort food, or food for dealing with stress or frustration)

_____ A thin person eating a luscious food, giving the impression that if he or she can eat it so can you

_____ Attributing positive characteristics to people who eat a particular food (they are fun, sexy, manly, and so on)

_____ Specials at restaurants, advertising a special holiday meal or a new menu item

_____ Symbols and brand names (such as McDonald's golden arches), which we react to automatically, even on a subconscious level

_____ Food names that include special adjectives to entice us, like "Flaky Southern buttermilk biscuits" rather than just "biscuits"

Now that you know your most significant triggers, pay attention to your reactions to them during the day. Instead of mindlessly reacting, choose your response to these media cues consciously and thoughtfully.

media triggers of mindless undereating or dieting worksheet

The triggers below typically try to sell you diet foods or products like exercise equipment. Ask yourself whether you are vulnerable to these triggers. Place a check mark next to the situations that apply to you.

_____ Ads that show the negative stereotypes often associated with someone who is overweight (for example, laziness or low intelligence)

_____ Plans that promise a quick fix for weight

_____ Products stating that you are smart if you buy them

_____ Products covered with labels like "low fat" or "low calorie" to suggest that they are healthy

_____ Ads that suggest that you will be happy if you are thin

_____ Ads that imply you should look a certain way, like a supermodel, and if you don't there is something wrong with you

_____ Ads that suggest you should be perfect or fix yourself to become that way at any cost

_____ Pictures that imply that if you eat this product you will be well liked or more sexually attractive

_____ Ads that place women as the object of beauty

Thankfully, there has been a recent push to make sure media ads don't promote dieting and starvation. For example, during Spain's Fashion Week, the fashion industry put their foot down: they didn't want to put models' health at risk. So, they required models to be at a minimum weight, a weight above the anorexia level on the body mass index. Thirty percent of the models were turned away for being too thin. Other fashion boards in various parts of the world are starting to consider following suit.

Change is definitely happening. Open a popular women's magazine and you won't be too shocked to find a growing number of models with a real woman's figure (curvy and not stick thin) in advertisements. Dove

> ## Mindful Eating Tip: *How to Be a Mindful Consumer*
>
> When you see a commercial, magazine article, or ad, try the following steps:
>
> 1. Use the Ten-Second Rule. Most ads only get a glance. Ordinarily, you might look at an ad for a split second, just long enough to see it and get the obvious message. Instead, look at it longer than just a moment. Place all of your attention on it. Absorb it.
>
> 2. Identify the obvious message. What is this trying to sell you?
>
> 3. Draw your *awareness* to the more subtle, underlying message (for example, "You will be sexier if you buy this").
>
> 4. Notice your first gut reaction to the ad. Does this ad include people with natural body shapes and sizes? Does it show people eating balanced meals? Or does it have airbrushed, emaciated models? How does it make you feel?
>
> 5. How is your initial gut reaction different from your mindful awareness of its obvious and implied message? Does the underlying message make you angry, irritated, or intrigued?
>
> 6. How can you continue to be more mindful of media triggers?

bath and body products are a stellar example of this change. They use women in their ads that represent the majority of society. Kudos to them! Other advertisers have taken an innovative approach. They sell their products based on the idea of promoting strength rather than slimness.

Men are by no means immune to the media's wicked body image tricks. Male celebrities' images in magazines are just as airbrushed these days. As we see the number of men struggling with eating problems and body image problems, we will continue to see this reflected in what we see in magazines, on billboards, and on TV. Male issues with body image and mindless eating have been severely neglected. Over the next few years, you will see resources like this workbook aimed at helping everyone, regardless of gender, eat in a mindful way and deal with a damaged view of their appearance.

The media sets the stage for mindless eating. The cultural messages you get every day are not just factored into the way you eat; they are evident in your speech. You can see how much you've internalized these messages by the way you talk to yourself and others.

mindful speech

My clients share with me the critical words they use to describe themselves: "fatso," "chubster," "thunder thighs," "pig." In counseling, we work on erasing the critical tape in my client's head, rewinding, erasing, and recording over it with more compassionate mindful speech.

We are all guilty of blurting things out before we have really thought them through. The extra words that spill out are mainly white-noise words that act as opinions or judgments. We don't need these words to get our point across or get the job done. Or, in our self-talk, we attach ourselves to words that bring us down. For example, you have the thought, "I'm such a cow—I can't control my eating!" and suddenly you find yourself repeating the phrase over and over again in your mind. You can't let it go.

When you speak mindfully to yourself and others, you sift through the vast number of thoughts you have. You stop the constant chatter in your head and slow down. Speaking mindfully is carefully selecting words that are helpful rather than harmful to your endeavors to eat mindfully. Words that are exaggerated, untrue, or judging impede the ability to be in the moment and move forward.

the mindful speech test

Bring to mind the following quote by Sai Baba: "Before you speak, ask yourself, is it kind, is it necessary, is it true, does it improve on the silence?" After your next conversation (in your head or with someone else) about mindless eating or your body image, recall what you said:

What did you say?

_____

_____

Was it kind and compassionate? Was it judgmental?

_____

_____

Was it true? Did it "feel" true to you but perhaps violate someone else's truth? Was it exaggerated?

_____

_____

Did it improve on the silence?

_____

_____

_____

What Is Mindful Speech?

Mindful speech is compassionate. It has empathy and is kind. Learning to speak this way requires a lot of work after years of critical self-talk. When people begin to use compassionate words, they often say, "But I don't believe what I am saying if I speak nicely to myself." At this juncture, that is okay. Keep bringing up compassionate words and use the basics of the mindfulness language you've learned in this book. Statements should be neutral, compassionate, and mindful. Remember that speaking mindfully is like learning a new language, such as Portuguese or French. At first, it takes effort to remember the new words, but over time it becomes second nature. Here are some examples of motivating and compassionate words and phrases:

- "It's really not that big of a deal. It's okay."

- "I'm not 'bad' for slipping up, I just need more work."

- "I can forgive myself."

- "I will pause and re-center so I won't be so critical of myself."

- "I need to dissolve my anger."

- "I don't need to judge myself. This isn't a courtroom."

- "If it were one of my friends, I would empathize with him or her."

mindful eating exercise: compassionate self-talk

Make a list of your own motivating and compassionate words and phrases:

_____

_____

_____

_____

Being in the moment with mindful talk:

1. When deprogramming your critical self–talk patterns, first notice *what* you say and *how* you say it. Do you have a typical insult for yourself? Is your tone sarcastic or scolding?

   _____

2. Then notice *why* you use the words you do. What function do these words play? For example, when you put yourself down, pay attention to the *outcome or purpose* of these words. Are you trying to punish yourself?

   _____

3. Do you say what you mean and mean what you say? Are you expressing what you are really trying to communicate? Think carefully about your real message.

   _____

4. Notice the impact of the words. Pay attention to how you feel and behave when the words are like a punch in the gut, compared to a gentle pat on the back. You ask yourself, "What impact does this statement have on me? Does it hurt? Does it motivate me to change? Is it true?" You will begin to see the outcome of the words. It's like watching a ball leave the pitcher's hand and noticing how it hits the catcher's mitt.

---

mindful eating exercise: rewriting the mindless script

What would you typically say to yourself? Write the uncensored version below.

Now, rewrite your statement to yourself, using mindful language and nonjudgmental, compassionate words.

Awareness of Toxic Table Talk

A frequent topic in therapy is how to work through some of the harsh words friends and family members have said to my clients about their weight or body. The critical (and sometimes cruel) words have adhered like superglue to their brains. "My grandmother said I was getting blubber thighs, and ever since I've obsessed about my weight," for example. The damage done by these kinds of harsh words is enormous.

Although it may be difficult to keep this in mind, know that the comments people make about your body say more about *them* than they do about *you*. People can't help but project some of their own weight issues onto others. If a friend notices an increase or decrease in your weight, this is typically because this friend is hypersensitive to changes in his or her own body and may tend to compare his or her weight to that of others. So take what people say with a grain of salt and remember that it is often, in part, a reflection of their own worries.

Further, compliments can be complicated: "You look great. Have you lost weight?" or "Wow. You look fantastic." These sound nice. However, people with weight issues may hear these compliments and twist them into backhanded criticism. They think, "So how terrible did I look before?" Or, they become terrified that they won't look nice and that people will judge them if they gain any of the weight back. Clients also say that compliments can bring up anger. If they are literally starving themselves, it is terrible for them to receive kudos for hurting their bodies. (The best policy is to avoid commenting on people's weight, whether your words are positive or negative. If you have to comment, say something like, "You've been putting a lot of effort into being healthier, that's great. I admire that you walk two miles every day!")

mindful eating exercise: mindless speech and toxic table talk ———

It is important for you to know how other people's words influence how you eat. Your task in this exercise is to pay attention to food talk. Notice what people *say* about food. Begin this exercise by thinking about your most recent conversations about food, weight, or dieting. Or wait until the next conversation occurs and examine it closely through this exercise. First record the date, time, and place the conversation occurred.

_____

Next, record exactly what was stated. What was the significance of the conversation to you? How did it impact you? Write about this on the line below:

_____

_____

_____

_____

_____

_____

Mindful Eating Tip: *Bond with Other Mindful Eaters*

Work on finding mindful eaters to dine with. If you can't avoid mindless eaters, then aim to notice their impact on you.

Can friends sabotage your mindful eating? They might. If you have a friend who is overweight, then your chance of also struggling with your weight increases by 57 percent, according to findings reported in the *New England Journal of Medicine* (Christakis and Fowler 2007). On the plus side, the opposite is true as well. People tend to eat better and manage their weight if a friend does so as well.

minding your surroundings

If you've completed this chapter, you've taken a good, hard look at your kitchen, pantry, and refrigerator. At this time, you are most likely feeling motivated to rework your surroundings to make them as mindful and peaceful as possible. You may have started this process by cleaning out your pantry. Maybe you tore up your old shopping list and created a new one, or perhaps you've taken a look at your bookshelf to see what you are reading about food. When you open up magazines or see commercials, you do so with a watchful eye. When you talk about food, you try to do so mindfully. You have taken some great steps toward making a home and work environment that supports your new mindful eating skills.

CHAPTER 8

nonjudgment

*Your worst enemy cannot harm you as much
as your own unguarded thoughts.*
—Buddhist saying

Emma battled with mindless eating for over ten years. She was tired of her weight issues and was feeling very depressed. Food dominated every thought, but her weight was out of control. Emma decided it was time she did something about this problem. She was ready and highly motivated—she knew she couldn't live like this anymore.

So Emma made an appointment to see her doctor, with the good intention of getting help. She wanted to know how to improve her diet. Once sitting in the doctor's office, however, she quickly made up another story about why she was there. Twenty minutes later, before she even saw the doctor, she walked right out without saying one word about her mindless eating. She had done a similar revolving-door routine about five times before this visit.

So many mindless eaters tell the same story. They really want help with mindless eating but are reluctant to ask for it. What stands in the way? Clients like Emma are often so fearful that their doctor or nutritionist will confirm their own self-judgments. Emma anticipated that her doctor would scold her. He would tell her how "bad" she had been by mindlessly eating—because that is exactly what she thought of herself. Fear of harsh criticism is enough to make mindless eaters avoid discussing the topic altogether. Of course, this kind of tongue lashing by care providers does happen occasionally (mostly as a projection of the health professional's own anxieties!), but not as often as people may fear. Unfortunately, this fear prevents many people from every broaching the topic that they so desperately want help for.

Sometimes it doesn't even take the judgment of another person to shut you down. Even your own self-judgment may have been enough to make you say, "I'll just deal with it tomorrow." Or, maybe you've wanted to just bury your head in the sand. Any number of defense mechanisms can spring into action when you feel judged. If this is hard to imagine, think about telling someone your deepest, darkest secret. It's likely that you will tell someone the truth when you aren't afraid you'll be ridiculed or criticized. You might even hide things from people, even your mother or a close friend, if they are disparaging. My clients talk about putting on a false front to avoid other people's harsh (and sometimes cruel) words or in order to appear as if everything is fine. In truth, you can only be honest with yourself and others when unkind judgment isn't involved.

Compassion and empathy are the remedy for judgment. They allow you to address tough situations and behaviors that need improvement, even when these cause you distress. All it takes is listening compassionately to your feelings. Put your inner judge and jury aside.

Focus on just describing the situation or problem. Notice the difference between thinking about yourself as "fat" and thinking of yourself as "overweight." "Fat" is a judgment. "Overweight" is a description. It's easy to beat yourself up whenever you slip up, by diving into a bag of chips or falling into your old mindless-eating ways. When you are compassionate with yourself, you are much more likely to address the problem productively than avoid it. Compassion helps you turn toward rather than away from uncomfortable situations.

In this section you will look at how to be compassionate and not judgmental toward your thoughts and feelings.

mindless inner critic

We all have a little inner critic that lives in our heads. My clients describe it in a lot of different ways: a sports commentator explaining the person's moves as they happen, a strict grandmother giving lectures and advice on dos and don'ts, or a nagging little voice. The inner critic is often the internalized voice of caretakers or someone who has been critical in the past.

This voice might also be called a "mindless critic" when these thoughts are automatic, springing to mind without any effort, or when the thoughts take place below your awareness. You are thinking mindlessly when you aren't really paying close attention to the thoughts, but they are influencing your reactions like a backseat driver.

Regardless of what the inner critic sounds like in your head, that voice is often full of judgments. The inner critic can also take on several roles, playing one or another depending on the situation:

- **The Judge** likes to find fault with what you do, is full of judgments, and is very critical of your actions. "I can't believe you ate that!"

- **The Punisher** is the part of your head that comes up with a penalty or retribution for what you've eaten. "No dinner for you because you messed up again."

- **The Fretter** second-guesses you for what you have eaten. "Is that okay to eat or not? I'm not sure."

- **The Partier** urges you to do it anyway and tells you that you are no fun if you don't. It talks you into ruining mindful eating. "Come on, what the heck. You'll start dieting on Monday."

- **The Wasn't-Me** denies what has happened or makes excuses. "But I couldn't help it."

- **The Threatener** tries to control behavior with threats and bargaining. "If you mindlessly overeat, you can't watch TV tonight."

- **The Danger Zone** feels afraid and overwhelmed. "I feel out of control!"

- **The Name Caller** uses derogatory terms. "How could you? You're so stupid!"

- **The Diet Book** tells you that you didn't follow the diet rules. "You shouldn't eat that. You blew it!"

The first step to being more compassionate is to just be aware of when criticism is happening. Just pay attention to it. Compassionately bring it to your attention by saying, "Oh, there is the Name Caller popping up in my head." At this point, just notice your mind saying, "Oh my gosh, are you stupid! You can't eat that!"

Again, thoughts affect your actions. If you don't take hold of and make friends with this inner critic, by welcoming it in and seeing what it is up to, it will take control. These kinds of critical thoughts produce a debate in your head, and the inner struggle takes you away from the moment. Notice how often the mindless inner critic enters. You may even want to write down what it says, or keep a tally of its comments. The next step, later on, will be to notice how that judgment could lead to a mindless eating action.

> ### Mindful Eating Tip: *Be Curious About Your Inner Critic*
>
> When you notice yourself getting hard on yourself for mindlessly eating, or your inner mindless critic speaks up, take a moment. See if you are experiencing a diet-related judgment. Are you breaking one of your old diet rules? Or is one of the thoughts listed above entering into the picture?

When you talk back to the critic now, use your mindful inner voice, or consciousness—your own little Jiminy Cricket sitting on your shoulder. This healthy, compassionate, logical voice encourages you to eat mindfully. The mindless voice will talk back, being critical, urging you to eat mindlessly, and it is often infused with guilt or emotion. Review a dialogue between the mindful and mindless sides. Imagine that you are at a party looking at a big piece of cake in your favorite flavor. You want a piece, but you are struggling with the decision.

Mindful Voice: I'm so full. Eating an entire piece of cake would not be mindful.

Mindless Voice: Don't you dare eat that piece of cake! You're so fat and don't need it anyway. Although it is vanilla cake with thick chocolate icing—your favorite.

Mindful Voice: True! But it's so sweet. It might even make me a little sick, since I'm already stuffed.

Mindless Voice: What the heck! It's a party. You have to celebrate. You can start again tomorrow.

Mindful Voice: What about just a little sliver? That way I could taste it but not regret it. It would still be mindful because I would not make myself overly full, and it would be polite to have some. I love vanilla cake; it's a party and I want to enjoy it too.

Mindless Voice: You don't deserve to eat the cake.

Mindful Voice:	Why not? Everyone else is having some.
Mindless Voice:	Because your body is not perfect. And, according to your diet rules, cake is a no-no, no matter what the occasion.
Mindful Voice:	So what? Nobody's perfect. And that is ridiculous; this is a birthday party.
Mindless Voice:	If you have one piece, you might lose total control. You will feel so guilty for the rest of the day.
Mindful Voice:	I am in control. I can have one small piece, and it won't make me lose it. If I eat one, I don't have to eat more. I am in control of my body and actions.
Mindless Voice:	If you let the host cut a piece, she'll give you a big slice. You know you'll eat every last bit.
Mindful Voice:	I'll just say to the host, "Oh, let me help you! I'll just cut a little piece. Thanks so much. It looks delicious. Chocolate frosting is my favorite." Then I can be in charge. Less is more, particularly with cake.

mindful eating exercise:
hearing but not heeding your mindless inner critic

It's important to really hear the critic's words. Actually, you can't turn them off. If you have tried, you know it isn't possible to control or get rid of these thoughts. The critic violates the mindfulness stance with words of judgment. When you hear yourself judging or being critical, simply acknowledge it: "Oh, there is my critic again."

Although you can't make the critic disappear, what you can do is choose not to believe, act on, or accept what the critic tells you. You can talk back.

In the space below, write what you hear the mindless inner critic saying (for example, "You're so stupid. You messed up your mindful eating again!"):

_____

_____

Now, write about what it means to you to not listen to or act on the mindless inner critic's words (for example, "I'm so used to talking down to myself that I hardly even realize I am doing it. I will try to recognize when my mindless inner critic is talking"):

_____

_____

If you were to talk back to the critic with your mindful voice, what would you say? (For example, "Stupid is a judgment. I can do better. It wasn't perfect, but I'm not always perfect. Sometimes I eat very mindfully.")

_____

_____

As you read this section, it's likely that you've started thinking deeply about how compassionate or terrorizing your inner voice is. Is it like an army drill sergeant? A comforting kindergarten teacher? Or somewhere in between? That inner voice likes to take charge and tell you what to do. Sometimes it is right on, and sometimes the advice is pretty misguided.

what is nonjudgment?

A nonjudgmental attitude is among the key elements of mindfulness and mindful eating. It's defined as the ability to see things as they are, without adding commentary or value judgment. Try for a moment to describe something without some judgment (words like "good," "bad," or "terrible"). It's tougher than it sounds. It actually takes practice. Whether you know it or not, you probably judge things a lot. It's difficult to simply describe an experience or thought without casting a judgment or analyzing it to death. People are particularly judgmental when describing their eating habits. For example, they might say, I ate a bad food—total junk," or "I was such a failure when I ruined my diet again."

It's Okay to Feel and Think as You Do

A nonjudgmental attitude allows you to welcome all your emotions and thoughts into your mind, even the ones that make you cringe. This will help you investigate and dissect them. When you allow everything in, you learn how your thoughts and feelings really work. As you get the hang of it, you will start to slow down the process. You will notice the event ("Oh, there is that thought again"), and you will notice the moment before you add a judgmental thought to it ("And there goes my mind again, wanting to put it all into a category of good or bad").

When you are nonjudgmental, you separate your reaction from the event that has happened: what is eating the cookie, and what is your *thought* about eating the cookie? You'll find that your thoughts and feelings, especially around food, are not a perfect reflection of what has actually occurred. Interactions with food are based on what you think and feel in that moment. Let's say you eat a nice juicy steak: if you are feeling good, you will enjoy it, but if you are thinking in that moment that you are fat, you might feel guilty or uncomfortable. As shown in this example, you may feel great or terrible after eating the same food.

nonjudgment and thoughts

In this section, you will learn how judgmental thoughts trigger mindless eating. It's likely that a pattern of thoughts clouds your mind and awareness.

When you are mindful, the goal isn't to get rid of painful thoughts. And, if you could get rid of them, you would have done so already. Instead, the goal is to understand how you think and to calmly notice your thoughts without reacting to them. You can have a thought without really believing it or following its instructions. Disobey the thought.

Many people get caught in the content of their thoughts. For example, when people have a thought like, "I'm so overweight and uncomfortable with my body; everyone is disgusted by it," they get sucked into an emotional hole of shame and anger. Instead, notice the *way* you think rather than the content of what's on your mind (for example, "I notice that I *think* about feeling heavy and fat whenever I have a hard day or I just ate something fattening"). It's a little bit like listening to the melody of a song rather than the lyrics.

mindful eating exercise: thoughts scale

Use the scale below the next time you eat. Or, choose a period of time and track the kinds of thoughts you have (such as judgmental or obsessive). Check in with the activity in your head frequently. What do you notice? What type of thoughts do you have? What makes you jump to different places on the scale?

Mindfulness of Thoughts Scale

10   One hundred percent of my thoughts are about food, my body, or eating. I cling and react to thoughts and urges. Obsessing. Dreaming about food or having a different body. Craving. Planning. It's very difficult to let go of thoughts.

9   Almost all of my thoughts are about food and my body. There's little room in my head for anything else. It's difficult to concentrate, read, or study. I react to beliefs and automatic thoughts.

8   Most of my thoughts are about food and my body. My behavior is strongly influenced by beliefs, rules, and food myths.

7   Some of my thoughts are about food and my body. I automatically believe my thoughts even if they aren't true. I have many "shoulds" and "shouldn'ts" that rule how I eat.

6   A little more than half of my thoughts are about food. Sometimes I notice when I am critical of myself.

5   About half of my thoughts are about food. Sometimes I am too busy to check in with my thoughts about food.

4   I check in once in a while with my thoughts. I am mostly able to observe my thoughts. Pondering what I would like to eat when necessary.

3   I'm carefully observant of my thoughts. When I have black-and-white thinking, I can consider the gray area.

2   I am able to step aside from thoughts. Critical or irrational thoughts don't rule my behavior. I allow thoughts to float by without getting caught in them. My mind is clear enough to focus on other things besides food.

1   I easily and effortlessly "let go" of thoughts about food and body. I can watch thoughts without getting caught up in them. Checking in occasionally with thoughts. Considering food options. Food is of some importance but not top priority. I can be mindful and concentrate on the task at hand without letting food dominate my thoughts.

An important benefit of mindful eating is the change in the amount of time you worry and think about food. Besides talking about wanting to lose weight, people express in counseling that they are sick of thinking about what they eat. They can't stand how much it is on their mind. It robs mindless eaters of the emotional room to think about or focus on anything else, particularly anything productive. They feel distracted, consumed, and less creative.

Given that you may want to think less about food, it's important to track the changes in your thought patterns. This is a great indication of healing. You will not notice your thoughts magically changing, but you will begin to see yourself starting to think less and less about it, gradually and slowly.

Mindless Thinking

People with eating issues are plagued with distorted thinking patterns. These kinds of thoughts spring to mind automatically (or mindlessly, with little effort). The consequence of mindless thinking is that it unconsciously affects your eating habits. Identifying the presence of these thoughts in your head is the first way to wrestle away their power.

Mindless thinking is based on extreme thoughts, sometimes called "black-and-white thoughts" (rather than thoughts with shades of gray). Eastern philosophy gives us the Middle Way. The Middle Way encompasses mindful thoughts, which are flexible and realistic but not extreme.

As extreme as they can be, mindless thoughts are also sometimes like background music: it's possible to not focus on them, allowing them to run in the background so they can fade out of your conscious awareness. But this doesn't mean they don't affect you. If the music (or mindless thought) is irritating, you might notice yourself getting agitated but not know why. When you become aware of the music (or thought), you might decide to change the channel. But if you don't notice it, you can't do something about it.

Identify which mindless thinking patterns you frequently lapse into. When a mindless thought happens, say to yourself, "That is an example of an extreme thought, and it is affecting what I am deciding to eat." Then, ask yourself what would be an example of a mindful thought, or the Middle Way. Below are a few types of mindless thinking patterns, along with examples of Middle Way thinking that might counter these thoughts. Below each type of thought, write down an example that you have personally experienced.

- **Extreme thinking** involves "either . . . or," perfectionistic statements. These thoughts don't allow any room for considering the middle ground or gray area. Examples include "I am totally in control" or "I am completely out of control," "I'm attractive" or "I'm ugly," "I am perfect" or "I am a failure," and "I am wonderful" or "I am terrible." The one people with eating or weight issues often use is "I'm fat" or "I'm skinny." **The Middle Way:** "I may not be happy with every aspect of my eating habits, but I am not always eating mindlessly and out of control. I am able to eat mindful portions on a good day." Or, "If I open up the bag, I have to eat the entire thing." This becomes, "If I open the bag, it doesn't mean I have to eat the entire thing. I can have a few."

_____

_____

_____

- **Worst-case-scenario thinking** is the overgeneralization of the potential outcome of the situation. "If I eat this brownie I will gain five pounds. Then, I'll never get a date." Sometimes it means using the word "always" or "never." These words overstate the effect when it is more likely to be "sometimes": "I always gain weight after going out to dinner" rather than "I sometimes gain weight." **The Middle Way:** "I will not gain five pounds from one brownie. I am striving to eat in moderation to help me feel better about myself. People like me for many reasons besides my body. If they don't want me because of five extra pounds, I am better off without them."

  _____

  _____

  _____

- **Overstating the facts** involves making sweeping statements that use one rule and applying it to a number of situations: "Being fat means you are lazy." **The Middle Way:** "Being overweight does not imply anything about my personality."

  _____

  _____

  _____

- **Turning the micro into macro** blows up the importance of an issue to a gargantuan proportion: "If I mindlessly overeat again, my life is over." **The Middle Way:** "I don't like it when I eat too much. It is hard on my body and I feel bad when I do it."

  _____

  _____

  _____

- **Abracadabra thoughts** include mythical and superstitious rules that seem to hold special powers: "If I have this diet drink, it will cancel out my mindless eating." **The Middle Way**: "How much weight I lose depends on a complex range of factors."

  _____

  _____

  _____

- **Putting on the blinders** means ignoring extremely important and informative information: "I don't see any evidence of physical problems, therefore the doctor is wrong; my eating is not harmful." **The Middle Way:** "I know mindless eating is not good for my body. Although I was uncomfortable when the doctor pointed it out, I realized the impact unhealthy eating can have over the long run and I am aware of the consequences."

_____

_____

_____

- **Overdoing it** involves having thoughts that overemphasize one's importance or relevance in the situation: "Everyone is looking at my body. They all think I am totally out of control." **The Middle Way:** "I am exaggerating. I am feeling vulnerable right now. A glance is just a glance. I am projecting my fears and judgments onto other people."

_____

_____

_____

- **Random theories** are personal theories made from a thought: "If I cut back on my food or stick to my diet, I feel relieved and in control, so I will never feel distressed or guilty if I continue to diet." **The Middle Way:** "There are lots of things besides dieting that help me feel relaxed and in control. It's not the only way."

_____

_____

_____

- **No-backup thoughts** are assumptions made without any concrete evidence: "People always like other people who are thin and eat mindfully." **The Middle Way:** "I would like this to be true because it would help me feel more in control. However, I know I don't like everyone who is thin; therefore this must not be true."

_____

_____

_____

From the examples above, take note of the type of thoughts you have the most frequently. Write down any thoughts that frequently sabotage your thinking.

_____

_____

_____

_____

The Middle Way: Now, try turning that frequent thought into a less extreme or less judgmental thought. Write it below.

_____

_____

_____

_____

self-sabotaging thoughts: dealing with "who cares?" and "what the heck?"

Notice when the "who cares" or "what the heck" thoughts pop up in your mind. These two phrases are responsible for undermining a lot of mindful eating! The "who cares" or "what the heck" approach is an example of all-or-nothing or black-or-white thinking; in essence, they are extreme thoughts. Let's say, you've created a food rule like "I can't eat past seven o'clock in the evening." You have made the decision to follow the rule to a tee. As a result, you might feel that if you break this rule you might as well break it all the way. But of course this isn't helpful to you. So, when the "what the heck" feeling creeps up, you can assume that something about that rule isn't working for you right now, and you can try to change your approach.

The goal is to move the decision *away* from either-or ("Either I follow the rule exactly or not at all"). Try compromising with the rule.

_____

1. Even though you may not want to, you have to pay attention to these self-sabotaging thoughts. Stop what you are doing. Devote your attention to working through thoughts mindfully. Say to yourself, "Oh, there is that feeling again." Write down your mindless thoughts, like "Who cares?" (For example, "It doesn't matter anyway. I will gain it all back anyway.") Then write a rational response to these thoughts (for example, "There is my brain self-sabotaging again. I will just focus *on this very moment*, not the past or the future but this very moment.") Take a deep breath. Focus for a moment on just your breathing. Try not to run away with any whirling thoughts going on in your head. Use this exercise to help anchor you back down into this moment.

2. In the space below, write about how you would feel if you were to follow the "Who cares?" approach.

_____

_____

_____

3. How can you turn a "Who cares?" into a mindful decision or compromise? Ask yourself, "What would make my response more mindful or middle of the road?" Maybe with the "who cares" approach you would eat three cookies, but a mindful approach would be to eat just one cookie. Below write about what would make this a more mindful decision.

———

———

———

Mindfully Watching for Self-Sabotage

I can't believe myself! I am so irritated. I have been eating mindfully for several weeks. It's been great. I finally found something that works for me. I feel full and in charge of my eating. What a huge change. Then, one day I just fell right off the wagon. I stuffed my face for an hour, completely throwing mindless eating out the window. I stood in front of the refrigerator and ate everything I could find. I felt terrible afterward. I could understand it if I enjoyed it, but I didn't. What happened? The funny thing was that I was totally aware of what I was doing. It was as if I wanted to feel bad again. Why did I torture myself?
—Amy

You were doing so well, getting so close to following a daily routine of mindful eating. You could see the light at the end of the tunnel. Now, out of the blue—wham!—you go right back to your old ways, with a huge mindless-eating episode. The crazy part about it is that you've knowingly sabotaged your own success. You think, "I set myself up! I knew I would definitely fall back into mindless eating!" You took the steps to make it happen.

Why do you engage in behavior that is sure to set you back? Sometimes your sense of yourself hasn't caught up to the new skills. You know *how* to mindfully eat. But your inner critic just won't allow it. The inner critic says, "Wait a minute, these aren't your old habits! Who do you think you are trying to change? You've always messed this up. Why get it right now?" As you can see, self-doubt and uncomfortable feelings creep up and push you back into old habits. If self-sabotage is happening, it means that you have some inner work to do in order to be mindful of old feelings standing in the way.

If it's not just an old habit coming back to haunt you, consider that self-sabotage might also be a way of controlling disappointment. If you don't expect to succeed and then you make sure you don't, you won't be surprised.

It's likely that you've gotten into a routine and unconscious pattern of self-sabotaging. Thoughts might include something like, "Oh well, I blew it anyway."

Behaviors of self-sabotage might include putting yourself in challenging situations with lots of triggers, like buying high-fat or high-sugar foods and putting them in your cupboard or going to a buffet restaurant (a sure trap).

minding self-sabotage exercise

Success and change can be scary, even when it is good. If you are struggling with self-sabotage, first gently acknowledge it. Then thoughtfully ask yourself the following questions:

1. What do you fear about success?

    _____

2. Do you feel worthy of getting what you want? Is being successful foreign to you? Or do you typically get what you want and have a hard time when you can't have it?

    _____

3. What other feelings do you associate success with? Pressure? Doubt?

    _____

4. Are you afraid that if you are successful, this will increase the pressure? Perhaps your expectations for yourself will increase and you don't know if you can meet them.

    _____

5. Are you worried that you will eventually disappoint yourself or others if you begin to do well and then slip up?

    _____

6. Are you worried that success will bring new challenges you can't face?

    _____

7. What behaviors, thoughts, and feelings do you engage in that lead to self-sabotage? Be very specific.

    _____

8. Are you uncomfortable with any new roles that mindful eating would require you to take on?

    _____

9. Are you struggling to let go of your identity or lifestyle that goes along with mindless eating (for example, someone who often goes out to dinner, or someone who is praised for his or her appetite).

    _____

10. If someone else was involved in sabotaging your mindful eating, first determine what kind of sabotage it was. Was it unintentional? (A well-meaning coworker baked you some brownies to thank you for working overtime.) Or was it intentional? (Your coworker noticed you were losing weight and became jealous. She brought in your favorite doughnuts because she knew you couldn't resist.)

_____

Acceptance can be helpful for self-saboteurs. First, recall that change is difficult. Then, use your nonjudgmental skills to listen closely to *why* your inner critic wants you to go back to your old ways. Is it in order to control disappointment? To protect yourself? To avoid a challenge? To stay with the familiar? To avoid expectations? To go back to comfortable, old habits? When you are mindful of the underlying reason, you can work on accepting the uncomfortable feelings that reason brings up.

minding what works

Have you ever gotten caught up in what you think you "should" do versus what really works for you? Think back to a time in your life when you ate the most mindfully. Maybe it was when you were working with a personal trainer or reading an inspirational book. Maybe you found that joining a group was helpful. It's important to know *what works for you* and capitalize on those successes.

finding solutions that work ————————————————

At what point in your life did you eat the most mindfully? Describe that time below.

_____

_____

What part of that situation increased your likelihood of success?

_____

_____

How can you use the information about your former successes now in your life?

_____

_____

_____

After you've identified what steps were helpful in the past, the next step is to visualize putting this behavior into practice again before you even try to take any kind of action. You'll find it helpful to do the mind work first.

Mindful Visualization

To accomplish your mindful-eating goals, you must imagine that they are possible. If you don't believe something can really happen, then it won't.

Most of my clients will say, "If I have a cupcake, I just can't stop at one" or "If I ate a cupcake I would feel so out of control and guilty." They can't even imagine being in control of their eating. They need to start with their *head* before they ever try to put the actions into practice with their fork.

Visualize yourself picking up a small piece of the cupcake, enjoying it, throwing the rest away, and walking away feeling satisfied. Picture every detail: the flavor of the cupcake and frosting, what the room looks like, how it smells, and the people who are there. Continue to visualize it over and over until it feels comfortable and you can see yourself doing it with ease.

Here are two of the benefits of visualization:

- Research indicates that if you can see yourself successfully eating mindfully in your mind's eye, you will increase your success of doing it in the real situation. Visualization techniques like this are often used to enhance an athlete's performance in his or her sport.

- Visualization changes your biological response to the sight of food. Imagine if I ask you to visualize biting into a lemon. When you visualize this the first time, you will notice yourself salivating and puckering. The sixth time you imagine it, for example, you won't have the same intensity of salivation. Your mouth might not even water at all. The same is true of foods that you tend to eat mindlessly. When you practice visualizing these foods, your body is likely to stop responding with the same intensity of craving.

mindful eating exercise: mentally making a path ⸻

Visualization makes a mental path. Let's say that it snows heavily in your neighborhood. The ground is covered with a foot of fresh snow. You decide to shovel the sidewalk. But you don't know where the sidewalk is because you can't see it. You would take a moment or two to visualize what the sidewalk used to look like. Then, in your mind, you outline a path that you are going to shovel. Making that path in your mind makes the job go a lot faster. You know which way to go. It helps you focus in the right direction.

Make a similar mental path before entering a situation involving food. For example, you walk into your office's lunch room and see a meat tray and a variety of snacks. Start by imagining what the lunch room looks like. See the situation in your mind. Imagine walking into the room, taking just one snack, and walking away. Watch yourself as you mentally enjoy the snack and perhaps talk yourself confidently through the urge for another.

Use the power of visualization to start working on a new behavior. For example, let's say one of your goals is to eat more mindful portion sizes. Before you go to bed each night, close your eyes and take a few moments to imagine yourself fulfilling this goal skillfully. See yourself in your mind putting smaller portions on your plate. Walk through in your mind what it would look like to eat until you are not hungry anymore but not too full. Write down this envisioned goal below to help you clarify what you want to start visualizing.

_____

_____

_____

_____

_____

_____

_____

The power of the mind can help you to prepare for stressful situations. It can gear you up and let you explore a mindless-eating challenge in a nonthreatening way. You can also use your mind to detach from the past, from beliefs that keep you stuck.

> **Mindful Eating Tip:** *Take a "Just Let It Go" Breath*
>
> As you take a breath, say to yourself, "I inhale a new, fresh perspective." As you breathe out, say, "I exhale all the 'shoulds,' or thoughts that no longer serve me." Repeat.

mindful attachment

Have you moved recently? The average person changes residences several times in his or her life, perhaps from parents' home to college to apartment to first house to a bigger home for a growing family. Each time you pack your bags, you get a true experience of the process of letting go and looking at attachment. As you sort through your belongings, it's likely that you ask yourself, "Do I really need this? Can I part with it?" People often come to realize that they have a lot of baggage and stuff. But throwing it out or giving it away can be agonizing. You might be surprised at how difficult it is to let go of that old lamp and those books you never look at.

We also get very attached to ideas, desires, and wishes. The struggle to let them go can be just as painful as letting go of cherished belongings. Perhaps you've become very attached to ideas about how you should eat, or have trouble letting go of past mindless-eating mistakes. Just like that old lamp, old ideas can be comforting even if you don't need them.

List the "shoulds" regarding your eating (for example, "I should be in control"):

_____

_____

_____

List the "shoulds" in your life regarding your body (for example, "I should be a size 8"):

_____

_____

_____

Come back to the metaphor of moving and letting go. Imagine putting these "shoulds" aside and placing them in a box. Visualize taping up the box and shipping it off, placing it in the trash, or simply leaving the box behind.

mindful perfectionism

Perfectionism and eating issues seem to go hand in hand. Whether the issue is a job, schoolwork, or their body, perfectionists have very distinct ideas of what they should be doing or what they must look like.

There are many good things about perfectionists. They work hard, do the job well, and are successful. The downside to being a perfectionist is that they set the bar so high that they are never happy with their accomplishments.

The trick for perfectionists is to set more *realistic* standards for themselves. A realistic goal is an obtainable outcome that you know you are able to reach without extraordinary effort.

perfectionist worksheet

Below are some of the key characteristics of perfectionists. Mark the beliefs that apply to you.

_____ I believe I am not allowed to make a mistake. I get very angry with myself when I do.

_____ I look for errors, slipups, or imperfections.

_____ I focus on the way things should be or what people expect of me.

_____ I don't like to do things that I know I won't do well.

_____ Nothing feels good enough; it could always be better.

_____ It is hard to feel satisfied.

_____ I desire to achieve.

_____ I have very high expectations for my friends and family.

_____ I use the word "perfect" a lot to describe things.

_____ I see the bad in a situation and have a hard time focusing on the positives.

_____ I can be judgmental of myself and others.

Write an example of one of your perfectionistic goals (for example, earn a huge end-of-the-year bonus at work by being the number one salesperson in the region):

_____

_____

Now, make this goal more realistic (for instance, make some extra income based on sales results: "I'd like to be number one, but I don't have to be"):

_____

_____

What perfectionistic goals do you have that pertain to your body and food (for example, to be a size 4 or always eat a certain way):

_____

_____

List a more mindful and realistic goal (for instance, to feel more comfortable in the clothes you already own):

_____

_____

guilt and mindful coping statements

Two monks traveling together reached a river, where they met a young woman. Wary of the current, she asked if they could carry her across. One of the monks hesitated, but the other quickly picked her up onto his shoulders, transported her across the water, and put her down on the other bank. She thanked him and departed. As the monks continued on their way, one of them was brooding and preoccupied. Unable to hold his silence, he spoke out, "Our spiritual training teaches us to avoid any contact with women, but you picked that one up on your shoulders and carried her!" The second monk replied, "I set her down on the other side, but you are still carrying her."

This story is an example of obsessing. Well after a regretful event such as an episode of mindless overeating has passed, it can be tough to mentally put the issue down. Like the monk in the story, many people can't seem to mentally let go of mindless-eating guilt. The guilt can last anywhere from seconds to days.

What do we typically try to do with guilt? We may:

Judge: "I am a terrible person."

Obsess: "I just can't stop thinking about how guilty I feel."

Self-criticize: "I can't do anything right."

Find excuses: "But I . . ."

Rationalize: "It's okay because . . ."

Assign blame: "It wouldn't have happened if you hadn't . . ."

Avoid: "I can't think about that right now."

Self-punish: "I don't deserve to eat."

Punish others: "I'm angry at you."

Not all guilt is bad. Sometimes, it is a gentle warning, a signal to watch out for similar behaviors ahead, a reminder to simply pay attention the next time you eat. However, when you place all of your attention on guilty thoughts, you are likely to get stuck and immobilized. You might find yourself replaying the event over and over like a broken record. So, instead of getting stuck in repeat mode, stop the record.

> ## Mindful Eating Tip: *Neutral Statements*
>
> Below are some examples of neutral comments. Repeat these out loud.
>
> - "I'm okay."
> - "I really do try hard; it's been a tough day."
> - "Next time, it will be easier."
> - "I'll try again."
> - "It's a struggle to be mindful."
> - "Everyone makes mistakes."
> - "I'm in pain, but it will pass."
> - "Being mindful is a process; it takes time."

How is guilt taking you out of the present moment? Ask yourself, for example, "Is it causing me to obsess? To avoid? What can I do in this moment that is different from what I did in the last? Am I engaging in the same behavior (like mindless eating) in this moment?" Describe below the mental and physical consequences of guilt.

_____

_____

_____

_____

Guilt is often the result of doing something that you believe is bad or has been labeled as bad, when you believe you should have been "good." This falls into the category of black-and-white thinking. Clearly, eating mindlessly doesn't mean you are a bad person, but thinking that way might become a habit.

Guilt Rocks

One of my clients said that guilt is like putting a rock in your purse each time you trip on one. You often take those rocks out and hit yourself over the head with them, rather than discard them or just notice them on the side of the path. You could instead choose to make your load lighter and your journey easier if you let go of each mindless-eating mishap and use it to learn how to avoid the rocks in the path of mindless eating.

The next time you are struggling with guilt, take just a moment and close your eyes. Imagine that you are holding a bag or purse. It is full of guilt rocks. Describe to yourself how heavy is it. Is it the guilt just slowing you down or weighing you down emotionally to the point you are almost paralyzed? Imagine what it would be like to take out a rock and throw it on the ground. Would it lighten your emotional load? Visualize using this rock not to beat yourself up but as a guide that teaches you how to avoid similar rocks. What did you learn from holding on to and then and letting go of this rock in your imaginary bag?

mindfully neutral

A big part of being mindful is to be neutral. Take the judgmental labels away and just describe the event as it is. Use descriptive words and adjectives. You also have to look at the context of the situation. In some instances, a big meal might not produce guilt, perhaps because you were starving before you began eating. However, the same meal might bring up a lot of guilt if you feel that you overate.

Describe the specific situation and the context of the event that prompted guilt.

I feel guilty because _____

_____

Make it neutral by just describing the event, without judgment. If judgment pops up in your mind, that's okay; just recognize it. Try not to judge yourself for judging (for example, "I feel so guilty for mindlessly eating those chips, and I shouldn't feel guilty!"). Instead, a more mindful response might be "Eating chips and feeling guilty are not good or bad behaviors, nor do they mean I'm a bad person. A feeling is just a feeling, not a fact. What I *mean* is that I feel too full when I eat extra chips." Write your neutral description of the event below:

_____

_____

_____

_____

_____

_____

_____

_____

mindful eating exercise: letting go of guilt —————————————

The most difficult feeling to let go of is guilt. Mindless eaters often hold tightly to guilt because they are fearful that if they let it go they will lose control again. A great way to work on letting go is to use visual imagery. Imagine tying the incident to the end of a balloon string and watching the thought (or incident) that is bothering you float up and away to the sky.

What did you tie to the balloon?

_____

_____

Why do you need to let go of these thoughts or feelings? Why would it be helpful to let go of them? (For example, you might write, "It's driving me crazy," "I can't move on with my life," "I have more important things to think about," "It's emotionally draining," or "There is nothing I can do about it.")

_____

_____

What do you fear will happen if you let it go? (For example, "It won't be the way I want it to be," or "I'm afraid I might do the same error again.")

_____

_____

_____

Guilt, judgments, and cruel self-talk are all part of the mindless-eating mind-set. Many people get caught in the belief that they just need to focus on cleaning up the content of their diet, such as cutting down on fast food and sweets. Although this is important, cleansing your thoughts is just as critical. The power of thoughts, particularly critical and negative thinking, is enormous. It can keep you treading water and not let you get anywhere. In the next chapter, you will learn about letting go of some of these negative beliefs and how to free yourself from other mental blocks that keep you stuck.

> **Mindful Eating Tip:** *Breathing Acceptance and Letting Go*
>
> On a breath in, say to yourself, "I have to accept where I am now." On the breath out, say, "I let go of the guilt."

CHAPTER 9

letting go

People have a hard time letting go of their suffering. Out of a fear of the unknown, they prefer suffering that is familiar.
—Thich Nhat Hanh

Letting go is like getting rid of your favorite sweater. You've had it for years, and it's out of fashion and worn out, but it's so cozy and comfortable. It's time to get rid of it, but there is a part of you that just can't do it. You've tried to let it go on several occasions, but you've fished it out of the trash each time. You think, "What if I can't find another one just as cozy and comforting as this?" Most of the suffering we encounter from mindless eating is the inability to let go of the desire for more and the tendency to hold on to things that are comfortable but aren't doing us much good.

If you are a parent, you have experienced hanging on and letting go. I often see new parents in my office who are trying to hang on to their old childless life. They miss the freedom they used to have, such as uninterrupted sleep and dinners in fancy restaurants. However, they experience more pain in trying to hold on to the old life. Running after a baby in a fancy restaurant is much worse than having a relaxed dinner in a child-friendly environment.

This chapter is about letting go of old habits—specifically, letting go of habits related to mindless eating, including dieting thoughts and a judgmental attitude. Passing up the urge to eat more food, even when it is really good, is a great place to start learning about the concept of letting go.

letting go of the desire for more food

Imagine for a moment a piece of hot-from-the-oven apple pie with a dollop of fresh whipped cream on top. Just thinking about it is enough to get your mouth watering. For mindless overeaters, the anticipation of taste can cause intense cravings.

Eastern philosophy proposes that suffering comes from desire, whether it is a longing for another bite of food or for material possessions. Once you obtain what you desire, you desire more. *Desire is without end.* Are you completely satisfied once you get what you want? Does buying the new car take away your desire for another? You can see how this directly translates into mindless eating problems. It's not the steak or chili-covered nachos at the root of the issue. It's the *desire* for another bite of steak or nachos. When you eat, you might find that you want the pleasurable experience to continue. The true challenge is to let go of something that tastes good.

If you are someone who loves the taste of food, and you tend to mindlessly overeat because of this love, remember that the ability to let go won't happen overnight. You will need to work on it each day. Just focus on continuing to go in the right direction. Your task is to focus on two things:

1. **Letting go.** Pain comes from attaching oneself to something good. Once you have it, you don't want to let it go. Notice that you feel intense discomfort when you are about to stop eating something tasty. Remind yourself, in this moment, "I am struggling with the issue of attachment. I'm attached to the taste and have trouble letting go. It's okay to grieve the loss of something good." Repeat this to yourself.

2. **Desire.** Pain also comes from desire. It's not really the food you want but the desire for the taste *to continue* that is the problem. Remind yourself, "Even if I have another bite, the desire will not be satisfied." Desire is an endless cycle.

If you were perfectly "in control," you'd probably be able to pass up every ice cream sundae and every extra slice of pizza. But, that isn't possible, nor is it even your goal. If this surprises you, read on.

> **Mindful Eating Tip:**
> *Letting Go When It Tastes So Good*
>
> Do a quick breathing exercise. Say to yourself, as you inhale, "I let go of the desire," and, as you exhale, "that has no end."

"letting go" of control

Sometimes letting go actually means having control.
—Jim Medlock

One of the benefits of being more mindful is gaining a sense of control—but not the kind of control you might wish for or imagine. When you are mindful, you don't gain control over the *outcome*; instead, you gain control over the *process* of what is happening. You are more in charge of your behavior and how you perceive the world around you, rather than being in control.

For example, people with eating issues often crave complete control, which they interpret as following their diet exactly. A bit of mindless eating isn't just a slipup; it feels like being out of control of their entire body. The person thinks, "How could I not follow my own rules about eating?" When we make control an either-or situation ("Either I am perfectly in control or I am completely out of control"), it's easy to find ourselves on the wrong side of the line.

When you let go of the need for control, you find freedom in the flexibility. For example, when you let go of the belief that you always have to be in perfect control and must never do any mindless eating, you have just taken a step forward. You have made a choice to be in charge of your beliefs. That is true control.

The reality is that you will have moments when you lapse. This is okay and is not the end of the world. You don't have to have perfect control to be in charge of your beliefs.

When You Hold on to the Need for Perfect Control	When You Let Go of the Need for Perfect Control
You become obsessed. When you keep seeking perfection in your eating habits, you ruminate and worry about it.	You are able to be flexible and give yourself permission to make a misstep.
You never find peace. You become plagued with the urgency to make it better now.	Things can become "good enough."
You become driven by a sense of failure.	You accept that there are aspects of mindful eating that you do well.

signs that it's time to let go of the need for control ———————————

Place a check mark next to the statements that apply to you:

_____ I think a lot about feeling out of control.

_____ I feel that I must handle every meal correctly.

_____ Any slipups in eating are unacceptable.

_____ If I don't follow the diet plan exactly, I feel totally out of control.

_____ I feel I must handle every problem that comes my way.

_____ I need to fix all of these things perfectly and as soon as possible.

_____ No one else can help me solve problems.

_____ I am the only one who does things "right."

_____ The people in my life need me to tell them how to get things done.

The Serenity Prayer, by Reinhold Niebuhr, reminds us how to accept unchangeable things in our lives. It's a saying about how to give up control. If it is helpful to you, say this poem to yourself:

God, grant me the serenity
to accept the things I cannot change,
courage to change the things I can,
and wisdom to know the difference.

Mindful Eating Tip: *A Letting-Go Breath*

When you are feeling out of control or you have the desire to be perfectly in control, use a breathing exercise to refocus yourself. As you inhale, visualize the air coming in through your nose. Say to yourself, "I accept that total control is an impossible goal." As you exhale, say to yourself, "Ah, the sound of letting go of control."

help! mindful urge control

Urges can seem like runaway trains—unstoppable once they get started. In fact, many clients feel that if they have an urge to eat (or restrict their eating) their only option is to act on it. My clients often say that they know they should not have engaged in unhealthy behavior, but it was as if their hands detached from their body. This is how powerful urges can be.

Consider the urge to scratch an itch. Let's say that scratching it would make it worse, by opening up a scab. You can use mindfulness to avoid acting on the urge to scratch:

- Just be *aware* of the desire to scratch. Notice where the urge is focused on your body. Is it on your arm? Focus your attention on what caused the itch (perhaps a fly landed on you).

- *Observe* the itch. Pay attention to how strong it is on scale of 1 to 10. Is it a continual urge or one that changes from moment to moment?

- Be aware of *judgment.* Notice critical thoughts like, "I can't stand this itch. It's terrible." Thinking negative thoughts makes it worse. Compassionately address it with positives, such as, "I can deal with this. I've experienced worse."

- Stay *in the moment.* Notice the changes in the intensity of the desire to scratch. In the first minute the urge might be a 10, but two minutes later it is a 9. The urge might be strong at first, but it will fade.

Similarly, you don't have to react to the urge to mindlessly eat or engage in mindless behaviors (or automatic behaviors) like binging, restricting, purging, or comfort eating. You can use these mindfulness steps to notice and accept urges, and let them pass. Next time you experience an urge to mindlessly eat or restrict your eating, follow these steps and use the following worksheet.

STEPS TO RESPOND TO URGES

- ***Be aware*** of the urge to eat (mindless eating behavior). When did it occur? What prompted it? Notice all the sensations and effects. Where is the urge located in your body? Your head? Your stomach?

- ***Observe*** the intensity of the urge. Label it. Is it worse or better than other urges? Place it on a scale from 1 to 10.

- ***Be aware*** of any judgments about the urge (or for even having the cravings).

- ***Stay in the moment*** as the urge changes from minute to minute. Hang in there. It might be moments or it might be days, but eventually the urge to act *will* fade.

---

mindless eating urges worksheet ———————————

Describe in detail the nature of the urge (for example, the urge to eat, binge, or diet).	How strong was the urge from 1 to 10? 1 = weak 5 = medium 10 = extremely strong	What did you do? Did you act on it? Were you able to let it go?	How did you feel afterward? Was it painful? Did you feel proud or ashamed?	List the mindful action to take the next time you get this urge.

mindful support

Other people can help us to let go, and finding good support is essential. However, getting the right kind of support, from healthy people, is often difficult because so many people have issues with food or their weight. Below are a few reasons people don't turn to their friends and family for help:

- They don't want to be a burden.

- They believe others would not understand. People who don't have food issues often don't "get it." Others can't separate their own eating issues from yours.

- They fear other people will try to coerce or control their eating.

As people get deeper and deeper into their eating issues, their relationships with others may become more and more strained. Food sometimes takes over as the number one relationship in their life.

How does this happen? Well, people who restrict food or diet often struggle with isolation. It is painful to eat with others, so they avoid it. Unfortunately, as a result they may lose sight of how healthy people structure their meals, and they also become very lonely. Similarly, mindless overeaters may also be fearful of eating with others. They are scared that other people will evaluate them as harshly as they do themselves. Sometimes they avoid going out to eat with friends, lie about what they eat, or consume food in secret. In order to eat mindfully, you need acceptance and support from loved ones.

Below, list the healthy people in your life that you could turn to for support:

List the people who are not supportive of your mindful eating journey (either overtly, by trying to sabotage your mindful eating, or covertly, by snide comments):

List the advocacy groups you can join or a therapist you can meet with (see the Online Resources section for information on how to find a group or therapist):

letting go today

If you find you have trouble letting go of the things that are bothering you, look for good sources of support.

Letting go is a challenging skill to learn. We often know what we want and have a hard time when things aren't the way we want them to be. You probably were surprised to read in this chapter that it's good to let go of the need for control. Until now, you might have been holding on tightly to the notion that you need to be in total control of your eating. But you now know that the need for control actually holds you back.

In the next chapter, you will learn the last skill of acceptance.

CHAPTER 10

acceptance

We cannot change anything until we accept it.
Condemnation does not liberate; it oppresses.
—C. G. Jung

What if you woke up one day and realized that you looked exactly like Abraham Lincoln? This is exactly what happened to Pete Raymond. In 1976, Pete trimmed his facial hair to resemble Lincoln's and entered a Lincoln Beard contest, where it was discovered that he looked almost exactly like the sixteenth president of the United States.

It's easy to imagine the internal struggle he must have experienced. Did Pete want to look like a famous figure from history? Probably not. In fact, he reveals on his website that it "took nearly twenty-five years for the idea [accepting that he looked like Lincoln] to take hold." This is similar to the struggle most of us have with our appearance. It's likely that you have a vision of how you want to look, and you are bound to have trouble accepting your appearance when it doesn't quite match your expectations.

The consequence of Pete's acceptance of this fact about his appearance was life changing. Not only did he admit to the uncanny resemblance, but he made playing the part of Abraham Lincoln his mission. He currently goes to schools and presents on Lincoln's life history, and he has modeled for the covers of books on Lincoln. He embraced his appearance as part of who he is and has done something extraordinary with it.

You too have probably wasted a lot of time fighting against some aspect of your body that is just part of who you are. Sure, you may not resemble a famous person from history. But it's likely that you have something that you appreciate about yourself. Perhaps you aren't crazy about the shape of your legs, but they make you a great volleyball player. Wishing for a different body keeps you from loving, nurturing, and appreciating your body as it is. Imagine how much attention you could focus on other things if you didn't worry so much about having a perfect body.

Learning to accept yourself is a key aspect of mindful eating. When you stop fighting with yourself about the way you think it should be and start accepting the way it is, you can start dealing with the problem in a healthy way.

what is acceptance?

Acceptance is defined as experiencing a situation and having no intention of trying to change it. If acceptance is tough for you, you aren't alone; it's difficult for many people. You know what you want, but when life doesn't match your expectations it can be pretty disappointing, even painful.

A situation where people learn a lot about acceptance is in a relationship or marriage. Inevitably, your partner is going to have some traits that drive you crazy, like leaving socks on the floor, watching sports obsessively, or spending hours shopping. You know that these characteristics are part of the package. Unhappy spouses are often those who believe that they can change their partner—a recipe for disaster. We all want to feel accepted for who we are; think about how you feel when other people try to change core parts of your personality.

We often feel that marriage and eating shouldn't be as painful and hard as they can be. They seem as if they should be easier. Similarly, one reason people have such difficulty accepting mindless eating problems is that they cause so much pain in their lives. It's totally understandable that they would have difficulty accepting them.

mindless eating and pain worksheet ────────────────

How much suffering does mindless eating cause in your life? It can take a significant toll on your self-esteem and daily functioning. Using the worksheet below, track the way your thoughts about mindless eating increase your stress and worry about it. Note the examples provided in the first two rows.

Date and event	How much did I fret/worry/suffer today, on a scale from 1 to 10	What thoughts increased my suffering?	How could I have reduced my suffering?
June 2: Mindless eating at work. A client brought in a huge tray of food.	I worried for about an hour about what I ate. My level of pain was an 8. I felt so guilty.	I really beat myself up. My thoughts made it much worse. I couldn't let it go. The mindless eating felt like a catastrophe.	Put the incident into perspective. It wasn't the end of the world. Use mindfulness skills to let go of worry and stay present in my work.
June 4: My friend said, "How can you eat that junk?"	I was so angry. I felt judged and embarrassed. I stewed about it the rest of the day. It was about an 8.	I interpreted what she said to mean that I was "wrong" or "bad."	I may have taken it too personally. She worries a lot about what she eats. I was projecting my own guilt.

Date and event	How much did I fret/worry/suffer today, on a scale from 1 to 10	What thoughts increased my suffering?	How could I have reduced my suffering?

acceptance and mindless eating

People are often confused by the notion of acceptance in relation to mindless eating. They don't distinguish between giving up and acceptance. But there is a distinction between accepting yourself as a person and accepting your behaviors. A parent may love and accept her child as a person yet still want the child to have fewer temper tantrums, put away his clothes, or pay attention. Where parents go wrong and leave permanent damage is when they believe that bad behavior equals a bad child. A healthier way is to love the child (faults and all) and work on improving the behavior. Children are motivated to improve when they feel loved. If they don't feel loved and accepted by the parent, they may think, "Why bother?"

> **Mindful Eating Tip:**
> *Acceptance Mantra*
>
> Breathe. As you inhale, say to yourself, "I allow it to be." As you exhale, say, "Just as it is."

Similarly, people with body image issues make the mistake of thinking that bad eating behavior (mindless eating) equals bad person. Instead it would be helpful to think "Accept myself, and tweak the mindless eating."

acceptance exercise: accepting the gift

First, imagine that you are at your birthday party, and you have received a gift. It is exactly what you wanted. Picture what this would be (but be realistic). Write down what this gift is.

_____

_____

Now, imagine that at your birthday party you are celebrating a friend's birthday as well. You can't keep this gift you love, because it was intended for your friend. And she has accidentally picked up the gift intended for you. You exchange it with her. Write down how it feels to let go of the gift you really wanted.

_____

_____

_____

The gift that was meant for you is something that you didn't really want. Describe a gift you recently got that you didn't really like.

_____

_____

_____

Consider what you could do with this gift. How would you make the gift fit into your life or be of use. For example, you might give the gift away. Maybe you hold on to the gift anyway in case it might come in handy someday. Write down what you could do with this imaginary gift.

_____

_____

_____

THE GOAL: Finding a use for a gift you don't want can give you inspiration. You can use this example as a guide for how to think about accepting your body. Your body is a gift. You don't always get the gift you want or ask for, but you accept it graciously and make it work or fit into your life.

minding your body-image history

Examine your body-image history. Understanding your past can help you understand how your body image, or your mental picture of yourself, developed and why it is so difficult to accept. Fill in the blanks below.

As a child, I felt _____ about my body. I described my body with words like:

_____.

As a teen, I felt _____ about my body. I described my body with words like:

_____.

As a young adult, I felt _____ about my body. I described my body with words like:

_____.

As an adult, I felt _____ about my body. I described my body with words like:

_____.

At this moment, I feel _____ about my body. I described my body with words like:

_____.

Growing up, my caregivers, friends, and family described my body with words like: _____

_____.

My caregivers, friends, and family currently describe my body with words like: _____

_____.

How does your view of yourself differ from how other people view you now and how they viewed you in the past?

_____

_____

Do you have difficulty "letting go" of your past identity or body image? Write about this below.

_____

_____

_____

This exercise may have given you some clues about why it is so hard to accept your body as it is. Throughout your life, your image of and relationship with your body will change. And part of accepting your body is being okay with the signals it sends you.

Acceptance of Hunger: Go Away, Hunger!

Imagine that your next-door neighbor is knocking on your door. You just got out of the shower and are wearing a robe, and you don't feel like answering the door. For a few minutes, the neighbor is knocking on the door lightly. You hope he will just go away! You deliberate. Should I open the door or not? Again, you ignore. What happens? The knocking gets louder and more impatient. The neighbor knows you're in there.

Finally, you realize that the neighbor is not going away. But the longer you wait, the more your attitude is going to change. When you finally do answer the door, after all that persistent and loud knocking, what condition are you likely to be in? Will you be frustrated? Angry? You might respond as if there must be an emergency.

This is similar to the way you may be answering your hunger. Your hunger gives you a little nudge and you just hope it will go away. The more you ignore, the louder the hunger signs become, and the more agitated you feel. The longer you wait and fight it, the more you are likely to eat out of anger, frustration, or urgency. Imagine the difference in your attitude if you were to welcome in the hunger as soon as it began knocking lightly. You could calmly and more rationally open the door.

"I can't stand feeling hungry!" The feeling of hunger is one that many of my clients profess to be one of the scariest and distasteful experiences. Jane, a sixty-two-year-old lawyer, said that if she could have one wish come true about her body it would be that the feeling of hunger would go away. When she felt hungry, she knew a decision was looming, and she started to worry about what to do about it.

It's important to accept the feeling of hunger. It's not going anywhere. Nor would that really be a good thing. Hunger plays a vital biological function, alerting you that your body needs fuel so it can keep going.

acceptance exercise

Repeat the following out loud:

I accept that hunger is a normal biological function. I will be hungry.

I accept that my body needs food to eat. Hunger is a necessary and important signal.

I accept that my hunger is sometimes scary.

I accept that it is difficult to meet my hunger accurately.

I accept that feeling hungry doesn't always mean I need to eat food.

I accept that I need to get to know the physical and emotional cues of hunger.

I accept that _____.

body acceptance

After many years of dieting and disliking your body, your approach isn't going to magically change overnight. It takes practice. Hang the affirmations below on a bathroom mirror, on a door, or in another visible place. Make a copy and put it in your purse or wallet. Read and reread them.

Body Acceptance Affirmations

- I accept that my eating and weight concerns are creating emotional distress, discomfort, and suffering in my life.

- I choose to accept my body and weight as they are at this moment.

- Committing to accepting myself is a choice only I can make.

- I accept that body obsession clouds my awareness and thinking.

- I accept that my genetic inheritance strongly influences my body shape and weight.

- I accept how important it is for me to eat mindfully in order to live a healthy life.

- To accept my body and weight does not mean that I am judging them to be perfect.

- Acceptance only comes from within myself. I can't seek it from the outside.

- I accept that my worth is not reflected in my weight and shape, but rather, my worth is determined by who I am as a whole person.

- Acceptance includes rejecting the cultural pressure to be perfect.

---

mindful eating exercise: write your own affirmations

Choose three things that you have difficulty accepting (about yourself, your life, your circumstances, your body, and so on) and need to work on. For example, I accept that mindless eating is a challenge for me and not for my husband. I don't like it, but I can work on accepting it. When I don't accept it, I obsess about how unfair it is. This isn't productive. I need to just focus on myself.

I accept _____

_____

_____

Betsy, a thirty-two-year-old nurse, explained how she obtained body acceptance. For years, she had wanted to be thin, pencil thin. She was never overweight, but at six foot one, Betsy was not the petite, tiny woman she dreamed about being. When she went to clothing stores, she found herself picking up clothing in small sizes. Daily, she wished she could squeeze into these clothes.

After spending a day with her dogs, she had an "aha moment." She explained that she loves dogs, all kinds of dogs. She said, "My wish to be thin is like my longing to be like a Chihuahua, tiny and petite. But I'm just not made that way. No matter how much I've wanted to be a Chihuahua, I'm not. I'm built like a Labrador retriever—and that is okay. The world has all different kinds of dogs. I wouldn't want my cocker spaniel to be a Chihuahua. I can't change my body. I need to accept who I am."

body mindfulness exercise: mindfully accepting your body ———

Stand in front of a mirror. Your task is to describe yourself without using judgmental language. Do not use words like "fat," "ugly," or "stupid"). Only use descriptive adjectives (such as "round shoulders," "flowing hair," or "knob-like knees"). First describe your hair (color, length, and texture). Notice the shape of your legs and shoulders. Describe your silhouette. Put into words some of the important functions that your body parts do for you.

mindfully feeling fat

Is "feeling fat" a trigger for you? Therapists will try to persuade you that fat is not a feeling. But, if it is not a feeling, then why do so many people say they feel that way? For many with weight issues, "feeling fat" is a difficult emotion to cope with. Your task is to dissect this feeling and understand where it originates. Be mindful of the underlying triggers.

body mindfulness exercise: what triggers feeling fat? ———

Is it a *physical sensation* that sparks your "feeling fat"? Do you feel fat when your pants feel tight, when your stomach is full, and so on?

_____

_____

Is it a *thought?* What thoughts or memories come up when you are feeling fat?

_____

_____

Is it a *feeling?* Painful or difficult feelings such as "I don't feel good about myself" often get translated to "I feel fat." What other feelings can you name that arise when you are "feeling fat"?

_____

_____

When you are "feeling fat," follow the steps below.

1. Identify what sparked your "feeling fat": a thought, feeling, or physical sensation. Identify the circumstances. Where were you when the feeling hit? What happened? Write about it here.

    _____

    _____

2. What do you typically do to cope with this feeling? Most people develop a plan (often an unrealistic plan), such as telling themselves, "I am never going to eat again," "I'm going to start my diet tomorrow," or "I'll skip a meal." People with disordered eating sometimes engage in very harmful behavior like restricting or purging to stop themselves from feeling fat.

    _____

    _____

3. What different response can you try the next time to cope with this feeling?

    _____

    _____

Instead of falling into your typical reaction next time you are feeling fat, notice and be present with the feeling. Read the following text out loud if you need to.

Focus on Mindfully Feeling Fat

Our natural human reaction is to act on an uncomfortable feeling immediately. Being mindful is the opposite of this—it is just observing. When you are mindful, you maintain a neutral stance while closely observing an emotion. You watch the feeling come, you watch its intensity, and then you watch it grow fainter until it is gone. Sometimes it may take only a few minutes for the feeling to fade, and other times it may take hours or even days. Don't panic. This watchful stance typically keeps the reaction in check, and you learn that what seems unbearable becomes bearable.

Feeling fat or guilty for mindless eating is a feeling that sometimes seems unbearable. As soon as the feeling arises, you don't know what to do with it and want to take action to get rid of it immediately. Sometimes this action is a behavior to make the feeling go away, like running. Sometimes it is self-punishment: "No dinner for me." Sometimes it is a thought: "I'm never going to eat again." Sometimes it is a feeling: "I am a horrible person." Your anxiety is slightly reduced because you have a plan to make yourself pay for it. However, these actions often make you feel bad about yourself (and may be difficult to accomplish, setting yourself up for possible failure) and start the cycle all over again.

mindful eating exercise: stay with the feeling ————————

The next time you "feel fat," just watch that uncomfortable feeling as if watching the waves in a bay rise and fall. Notice the feeling or guilt rising within you. Pay attention to the intensity of it. Take note of how long it takes to fade, but hang in there until it's gone. Try to hold off on reacting to the feeling. Distract yourself. Get out of the house. Call someone. Read this book again. If you interrupt the feeling, sometimes it fades a lot faster than you think. Respond mindfully by closely watching and knowing what prompted this feeling.

self-image and state of mind

> *When I am angry or tired, I am not a rational person. I look in the mirror and can't find a single thing I like about myself. I decide to punish myself with salad. But, when I'm well rested and after a fun night out, I feel okay. I don't make death threats to my diet. It's interesting how my state of mind changes the way I look at things.*
> —Rachel

In Eastern philosophy, there is a story about a monk who did not own a mirror. He didn't need one. Each day the monk got up and looked in a pot of water to see his reflection. Typically, the placid water in the bucket gave an accurate reflection of his face. But one day, when he looked into the pot, the water was covered with moss and water plants. When he gazed in the pot, he was shocked. He didn't see the reflection he expected. It was severely distorted. His features were muddled up and altered by the stringy moss. Imagine his reaction if he believed that the moss-covered reflection were an accurate picture of himself. What if he didn't realize that what was being reflected back to him was altered by the plants?

The moss is a good metaphor for the crud that grows on our mind when we start looking at ourselves through the eyes of the media and society. It's hard to accurately see and accept ourselves as we are. Like the monk, we believe our eyes, even though our vision is clouded .

There are a few different versions of this story, with several types of buckets the monk peeks into:

A busy mind: A monk looked into a pot filled with red, blue, orange, and green water. His reflection was distorted by the swirling colors.

How does your busy mind affect how you see your image and your body? Write about it below.

_____

_____

An angry mind: A monk looked into a pot of still water. Then he placed it over a fire, and it began to boil.

How does your angry mind affect how you see your self-image and your body?

_____

_____

Obsessing about the past: A monk looked into a pot of water that had been blown about by the wind; the old muck and mud that had been sitting at the bottom of the bucket had been stirred up.

How does your reminiscing mind affect how you see your image and your body?

_____

_____

_____

mindful acceptance

For after all, the best thing one can do when it's raining is to let it rain.
—Henry Wadsworth Longfellow

Acceptance is the last skill presented in this book. This is not because it is the most or least important. It was placed here because it is a good summary of the other skills. Accepting yourself, flaws and all, is also a good way to get started and a concept to come back to when you find yourself struggling. Acceptance is a mind-set. It's an important backdrop for being successful in mindful eating. Once you've accepted that mindless eating is a problem, you can then begin to find a way to work with that reality.

Longfellow got it right. Say you've planned a picnic, but it has begun to rain. You stew about the rain for a while, wishing it wasn't happening. Maybe you even rant and rave about it ruining your picnic. "It isn't fair! Why now?" You pace back and forth, hoping it will stop.

Once you've accepted that it's raining, you prepare yourself to deal with that fact. You might reschedule, or, move the picnic indoors. Perhaps you get a very large umbrella. But until you take that emotional step of letting go of what you wanted, nothing can change.

After reading this section, you may still be struggling a bit with this concept. Acceptance can take some time. What is most important is that you understand is that it is an integral part of how you approach mindful eating.

In the next chapter, we will cover just a few more issues that frequently come up when people are working on mindful eating.

CHAPTER 11

mindful eating review

Congratulations! You've successfully learned the ins and outs of mindful eating skills. Getting to this chapter means you have made a significant investment in your health and emotional well-being. How do you feel? I hope you are proud of the progress you've made and will keep going. You like how much knowledge you've gained about yourself. And you have a good handle on the factors that formerly stood between you and a mindful relationship with food.

The following pages will help you review what you've learned. Start by answering the questions. This will guide you as you put it all together. It can also test your knowledge, so you can see how much you've learned. One of the most important worksheets in this section covers relapse factors, the triggers that could send you heading right back to your old ways. When you know yourself really well, you will be able to clearly identify the factors that prompt mindless eating.

This chapter also includes a brief summary of the seven skills that you can copy and hang up. Place copies of the summary in locations you frequently see, like a bathroom door or kitchen cabinet. Posting the summary sheets near food will remind you to use these skills in situations that require you to ask, "Do I eat that or not?"

eating mindfully review questions

How would you describe your mindless eating habits (dieting, overeating, undereating, chaotic eating, or a combination)?

_____

_____

The foods you eat the most mindlessly:

_____

_____

The places you eat the most mindlessly:

_____

_____

You are best able to eat mind*fully* when you:

_____

_____

You tend to eat while multitasking when you are doing the following (for example, driving, talking, making dinner, working at your desk):

_____

_____

What you cling to that causes you a sense of unhappiness (for example, the desire to be a certain size, not wanting to change your eating habits, wishing it were easier) is:

_____

_____

You turn toward or away from food for comfort when you're feeling:

_____

_____

When you are mindful of your body, your body tells you that you are hungry by:

_____

_____

When you eat mind*fully*, your body's reaction is:

_____

_____

When you eat mind*lessly* your body's reaction is:

_____

_____

What you have learned about your thoughts is that you do the following (for example, have difficulty letting go of your thoughts without reacting to them, you are very critical of yourself, or need to work on being more compassionate to yourself and others):

_____

_____

What you have the most trouble accepting about yourself and your body is:

_____

_____

_____

mindless eating relapse prevention

A student went to his meditation teacher and said, "My meditation is awful! I'm so distracted, or my legs ache. I'm constantly falling asleep. It's just terrible!"

"It will pass," the teacher said.

A week later, the student came back to his teacher and said, "My meditation is wonderful! I feel so aware, so peaceful, so alive! It's just wonderful!"

"It will pass," the teacher replied.

As illustrated in this story, even if you've developed extraordinary mindful eating skills, at some point it will pass. You'll have your good days and you'll have your bad days. Even if you initially thought you'd pass this section up, the following relapse prevention worksheet is one of the most important worksheets you can complete. Do it today while you are doing well and *before* you have a relapse. Plan ahead!

The most important thing to remember is that you will experience a minor relapse or bout of mindless eating from time to time. Think of it as hitting a pothole in a road. You don't expect them, but every road has at least a few. Some are deeper and harder to get out of, and some just jolt us a little. When you encounter one, a minor relapse will require just a few tweaks, but a major one might mean starting over with this book or contacting a therapist.

When you need to get back on track, think about making a mindful U-turn. When you miss your exit, you simply find the next place to make a U-turn and get right back on track. It doesn't mean the trip is over; you just have to reorient and find the way again.

mindless eating relapse prevention worksheet ——————

The most important question you can ask yourself is the following:

What is most likely to prompt a mindless eating relapse? What circumstances (such as stress, the presence of food, or a relationship problem) would *trigger* it?

_____

_____

What factors make you vulnerable to relapse? (Examples might include being tired or lonely, eating in a Mexican restaurant, drinking alcohol, eating with mindless eaters, or feeling that you have messed up.)

_____

_____

What are the signs of a minor relapse? How would you know if you were experiencing a slight relapse? (Signs of a minor relapse could include having judgmental thoughts, leaning on food rules, taking mindless bites, or zoning out with food.)

1. _____

2. _____

3. _____

What are the signs of a major relapse? What behaviors are red flags of a major problem? (Perhaps you're feeling out of control, and unable to let go or work through cravings.)

1. _____

2. _____

3. _____

Mindful action plan: How to make your U–turn. What do you need to do to get back on track immediately? (Perhaps you might try getting out this workbook, reading, or going shopping mindfully.)

_____

_____

Mapping it out. What will you do if you are faced with this trigger again? (Choose a different restaurant, politely decline when offered the food, work mindfully through the craving, or get out of the house when bored to avoid using food as entertainment.)

_____

_____

_____

summary: mindful eating principles

This page summarizes the main principles outlined in *Eat, Drink, and Be Mindful*. Again, these are tips for the *way* you eat, not *what* you eat. The better handle you have on what motivates you to eat, the more mindfully you will approach meals and snacks.

- **Be Mindfully Aware:** Change nothing at first. Just be more aware. To raise your awareness, keep a mindful food journal. Make each bite a mindful bite. Smell. Feel. Look. Savor. Really taste.

- **Observe Your Body:** Slow down. Use a very deep breath as an anchor to pull you back into the moment. Put the fork on the table between bites. To find a balance between eating too much and too little, ask yourself, "How hungry am I on a scale from 1 to 10?"

- **Shift out of Autopilot:** Whenever you eat, ask yourself, "Am I eating out of habit or hunger? Am I eating mindfully? Make eating a conscious decision, rather than going through the motions.

- **Be Mindful of the Environment:** Notice how your eating habits shifts from place to place. Clean out your pantry. Put healthy foods in a highly visible place, and place trigger foods out of sight.

- **Be in the Moment:** Avoid multitasking while you eat. Turn off the TV. Put down the magazine. When you eat, just eat. Keep your mind at the table.

- **Practice Nonjudgment:** Speak mindfully. Be aware of critical thoughts about your habits or body. Move away from rigid food rules and use your mindful instincts. Food isn't "good" or "bad"; it's just food.

- **Let Go:** Let go of expectations for your body. Work on letting hurtful thoughts and emotional urges to eat go by without reacting to them. *Respond*, rather than *react*, mindfully to food cravings. The fact that you have a thought, feeling, or craving doesn't mean that you have to act on it or that it is true.

- **Practice Acceptance:** Adopt an attitude of "It is what it is." When you accept who you are—your body and hunger as it is—you stop punishing yourself with starvation diets and you no longer stew about the problem. Notice when you dwell. Start taking action by accepting the moment just as it is.

best wishes on your mindful eating journey

The mindfulness skills offered in this book may seem challenging, but they should help you on your journey toward eating mindfully. Remember, eating mindfully *is* a journey. It takes practice, and you shouldn't be surprised if you slip up from time to time. The key is not to give up when you stumble. Be kind to yourself, and let go of guilt. Use your mistakes to mindfully begin again.

Warmly,

Dr. Susan Albers

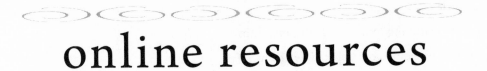

online resources

mindfulness websites

The following websites contain useful information about mindfulness:

www.eatingmindfully.com

http://studenthealth.missouri.edu/MPC/mpc.htm

www.mindfuleating.net

www.mindlesseating.org

www.emindful.com

www.mindfuleating.org

www.mindfulnessdc.org/mindfulclock.html

www.bangor.ac.uk/imscar/mindfulness/

www.umassmed.edu/cfm/mbsr/

www.mindfuleatingforlife.com

www.insightmeditationcenter.org

www.towson.edu/counseling/mindfulness.asp

www.mindfulnesstapes.com

www.jeanfain.com

www.marc.ucla.edu/

www.dukeintegrativemedicine.org/

mindful breathing exercises

Consult any of the following websites for mindful breathing exercises that are available for downloading:

www.marc.ucla.edu/

http://studenthealth.missouri.edu/MPC/mpc.htm

www.allaboutdepression.com/relax/index.html

nutrition websites

The websites below offer helpful information about nutrition and healthy eating:

www.nutrition.gov

www.eatright.org

www.healthyeating.net

www.hsph.harvard.edu/nutritionsource

www.nutritionexplorations.org (for parents)

eating issues websites

Visit any of the following websites for information about eating issues:

www.nationaleatingdisorders.org

www.anred.com/nes.html

www.edreferral.com

www.something-fishy.org

www.webmd.com

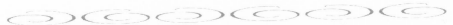

references

Allison, K. C., A. J. Stunkard, and S. L. Their. 2004. *Overcoming Night Eating Syndrome: A Step-by-Step Guide to Breaking the Cycle.* Oakland, CA: New Harbinger Publications.

Baer, R. A. 2003. Mindfulness training as a clinical intervention: A conceptual and empirical review. *Clinical Psychology: Science and Practice* 10 (2):125–43.

Baer, R. A., S. Fischer, and D. B. Huss. 2005a. Mindfulness and acceptance in the treatment of disordered eating. *Journal of Rational-Emotive and Cognitive-Behavior Therapy* 23 (4):281–300.

———. 2005b. Mindfulness-based cognitive therapy applied to binge eating: A case study. *Cognitive and Behavioral Practice* 12 (3):351–58.

Bellisle, F., and A. Dalix. 2001. Cognitive restraint can be offset by distraction, leading to increased meal intake in women. *American Journal of Clinical Nutrition* 74 (2):197–200.

Brown, K. W., R. M. Ryan, and J. D. Creswell. 2007. Mindfulness: Theoretical foundations and evidence for its salutary effects. *Psychological Inquiry* 18 (4):211–37.

Christakis, N. A., and J. H. Fowler. 2007. The spread of obesity in a large social network over thirty-two years. *New England Journal of Medicine* 357 (4):370–79.

Davidson, R., J. Kabat-Zinn, J. Schumacher, M. Rosenkranz, D. Muller, S. Santorelli, F. Urbanowski, A. Harrington, K. Bonus, and J. Sheridan. 2003. Alterations in brain and immune function produced by mindfulness meditation. *Psychosomatic Medicine* 65:564–70.

DiBonaventura, M., and G. B. Chapman. 2008. The effect of barrier underestimation on weight management and exercise change. *Psychology, Health, and Medicine* 13 (1):111–22.

Gore, S., J. Foster, V. Dillo, K. Kirk, and D. S. West. 2003. Television viewing and snacking. *Eating Behaviors* 4:399–405.

Grodstein, F., Levine, R., Spencer, T., Colditz, G.A., Stampfer, M.J. 1996. Three-year follow-up of participants in a commercial weight loss program: can you keep it off? *Archives of Internal Medicine.* 156(12): 1302.

Hollis, Jack, F., Christina M. Gullion, Victor J. Stevens, Phillip J. Brantley, Lawrence J. Appel, Jamy D. Ard, Catherine M. Champagne, et al. 2008. Weight loss during the intensive intervention phase of the weight-loss maintenance trial. *American Journal of Preventive Medicine* 35(2):18-126.

Kabat-Zinn, J. 1990. *Full Catastrophe Living: Using the Wisdom of Your Body and Mind to Face Stress, Pain, and Illness.* New York: Delta Trade Paperbacks.

Kalm, L., and L. M. Semba. 2005. They starved so that others be better fed: Remembering Ancel Keys and the Minnesota Experiment. *Journal of Nutrition* 135:1347–52.

Kristeller, J. L., R. A. Baer, and R. Quillian-Wolever. 2006. Mindfulness-based approaches to eating disorders. In *Mindfulness-Based Treatment Approaches,* edited by R. A. Baer. Oxford, UK: Academic Press (Elsevier).

Kristeller, J. L, and B. Hallett. 1999. An exploratory study of a meditation-based intervention for binge eating disorder. *Journal of Health Psychology* 4 (3):357–63.

Levitsky, D., and T. Youn. 2003. The more food young adults are served, the more they overeat. *Journal of Nutrition* 134:2546–49.

Linehan, M. M. 1993. *Skills Training Manual for Treating Borderline Personality Disorder.* New York: Guilford Press.

Linehan, M. M., H. Schmidt, J. C. Craft, J. Kanter, and K. A. Comtois. 1999. Dialectical behavior therapy for patients with borderline personality disorder and drug dependence. *American Journal of Addictions* 8:279–92.

Palmer, R. L., H. Birchall, S. Damani, N. Gatward, L. McGrain, and L. Parker. 2003. A dialectical behavior therapy program for people with an eating disorder and borderline personality disorder—description and outcome. *International Journal of Eating Disorders* 33 (3):281–86.

Prinz, P. 2004. Sleep, appetite, and obesity—What is the link? *Public Library of Science Medicine,* December 7. 1 (3):e61. http://medicine.plosjournals.org/perlserv/?request=get-document&doi=10.1371/journal.pmed.0010061.

Prochaska, J., J. Norcross, and C. DiClemente. 1994. *Changing for Good: A Revolutionary Six-Stage Program for Overcoming Bad Habits and Moving Your Life Positively Forward.* New York: Avon.

Proulx, K. 2008. Experiences of women with bulimia nervosa in a mindfulness-based eating disorder treatment group. *Eating Disorders* 16 (1):52–72.

Rolls, B. 2005. *The Volumetrics Eating Plan: Techniques and Recipes for Feeling Full on Fewer Calories.* New York: HarperCollins.

Safer, D. L., T. J. Lively, C. F. Telch, and W. S. Agras. 2002. Predictors of relapse following successful dialectical behavior therapy for binge eating disorder. *International Journal of Eating Disorders* 32 (2):155–63.

Safer, D. L., C. F. Telch, and W. S. Agras. 2001a. Dialectical behavior therapy for bulimia nervosa. *American Journal of Psychiatry* 158:632–34.

———. 2001b. Dialectical behavior therapy for bulimia nervosa: A case study. *International Journal of Eating Disorders* 30:101–6.

Shapiro, S. L., R. R. Bootzin, A. J. Figueredo, A. M. Lopez, and G. E. Schwartz. 2003. The efficacy of mindfulness-based stress reduction in the treatment of sleep disturbance in women with breast cancer: An exploratory study. *Journal of Psychosomatic Research* 54:85–91.

Smith, B. W., B. M. Shelley, L. Leahigh, and B. Vanleit. 2006. A preliminary study of the effects of a modified mindfulness intervention on binge eating. *Complementary Health Practice Review* 11 (3):133–43.

Taheri, S. 2006. The link between short sleep duration and obesity: We should recommend more sleep to prevent obesity. *Archives of Disease in Childhood* 91 (11):881–84.

Teasdale, J. D., Z. V. Segal, J. M. G. Williams, V. A. Ridgeway, J. M. Soulsby, and M. A. Lau. 2000. Prevention of relapse/recurrence in major depression by mindfulness-based cognitive therapy. *Journal of Consulting and Clinical Psychology* 68:615–23.

Wansink, B. 2006. *Mindless Eating : Why We Eat More Than We Think.* New York: Bantam.

Wansink, B., and M. M. Cheney. 2005. Super bowls: Serving bowl size and food consumption. *Journal of the American Medical Association* 293 (13):1727–28.

Warne, James P., and Mary F Dallman. 2007. Stress, diet, and abdominal obesity: Y? *Nature Medicine.* 13(7):781-783P.

Wilson, G. T. 1996. Acceptance and change in the treatment of eating disorders and obesity. *Behavior Therapy* 27:417–39.

Wiser, S., and C. F. Telch. 1999. Dialectical behavior therapy for binge eating disorder. *Journal of Clinical Psychology* 55:755–68.